SPANLINGO

SPANISH TO GO

For DENTISTS

&

DENTAL PROFESSIONALS

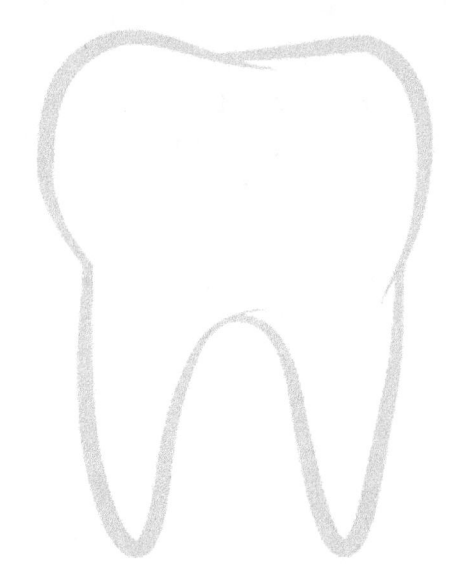

PATILIS

IN LOVING MEMORY OF MY FATHER, ANDREW PATILIS

Dear Dad,
This book is dedicated to you, with my deepest love and respect for the selfless sacrifices that you made for your family. You worked countless hours to make sure that your children would have the education and opportunities that were not availed to you.
Andrew Patilis, my dad, my hero. Not like the ones in the movies. A real life hero, who sacrificed his own dreams so that his children would have a better life. Your love for your family knew no bounds. Your family was your core and you led by love and example.
May you Rest in Peace in Heaven.

INDEX

DIRECTIONS TO THE PATIENT-DIRECCIONES AL PACIENTE

Traffic Signs→ Señales de tráfico

Turn to the right. → Doble a la derecha.	Turn to the left. Doble ala izquierda. →	Go straight ahead. → Vaya derecho.	Yield. → Ceda el paso.	Cross the street. → Cruce la calle.	Stop sign → el signo de alto /señal de stop
Turn right at the traffic light. → Gire a la dere-cha en el semáforo.	Turn left at the traffic light. → Gire a la izqui-erda en el semáforo.	One Way → Una vía	No Parking → Prohibido estacionarse	Speed Limit → Límite de velocidad	U-Turn → Hacer una vuelta en U

KEY DIRECTION WORDS

DIRECTION VERBS & INSTRUCTIONS TO PATIENT

Avenue → la avenida	North → norte	Cross → Cruzar	Cruce…
Block → la cuadra	Northwest → noroeste	Go towards → Ir hacia	Vaya hacia…
Corner → la esquina	Northeast → noreste	Go through → Atravesar	Atraviese…
Intersection → cruce	South → sur	Go past → Pasar al lado	Pase al lado…
Roundabout → la glorieta, el redondel	Southwest → suroeste	Turn → Doblar	Doble…
	Southeast → sureste	Turn around → Dar la vuelta	Dé la vuelta…
Sidewalk → la banqueta	East → este		Sálgase de la autopista…
Sign → el rótulo	West → oeste	Turn off the highway → Salirse de la autopista	
Street → la calle			
Traffic light → el semáforo			

DENTAL OFFICE BUILDING	PARTS OF A DENTAL OFFICE
The entrance→ la entrada	Central Sterilization→ la sala de esterilización
The exit→ la salida	Dental Laboratory → el laboratorio dental
The parking→ el estacionamiento	Dentist's Office→ la oficina del dentista
The elevator→ el ascensor	Dental staff lounge → la sala del personal dental
The staircase → la escalera	Operating Room→ la sala de operaciones
The receptionist→ el / la recepcionista	Reception Area→ la recepción
	Storage area→ el almacén
	Waiting Room→ la sala de espera

DENTAL PROFESSIONALS →PROFESIONALES DENTALES	DENTAL SPECIALTIES→ ESPECIALIDADES EN LA ODONTOLOGIA
	Cosmetic dentistry → la odontología cosmética
Dental Assistant→ el/la asistente dental	Dental anesthesiology → la anestesiología dental
Dental Technician→ el/la técnico,a dental	Endodontics → la endodoncia
Dentist→ el/la dentista	Forensic odontology → laodontología forense
Endodontist/root canal specialist→ el/la endodontista /el/la especialista en conductos radiculares	Geriatric dentistry→ la odontología geriátrica
Hygienist→ el/la higienista	Implant dentistry→ la implantología
Implant Specialist→ el/la especialista de implantes	Oral pathology→ la patología bucal
Orthodontist→ el/la ortodoncista	Oral & maxillofacial surgery → la cirugía oral o maxilofacial
Oral Surgeon→ el/la cirujano,a oral	Orthodontics →la ortodoncia
Pediatric Dentist→ el/la odontopediatra or el/la dentista pediátrico,a	Pediatric dentistry→ la odontopediatria
Periodontist→ el/la periodoncista or el/la especialista en encías	Periodontics →la periodoncia
Prosthodontist→el/la prostodoncista	Preventative dentistry → la odontología preventativa
	Prosthodontics →la prostodoncia

Tools and Equipment

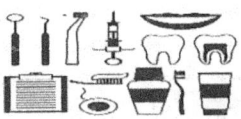

Dentist Chair & Parts La silla dental y sus partes

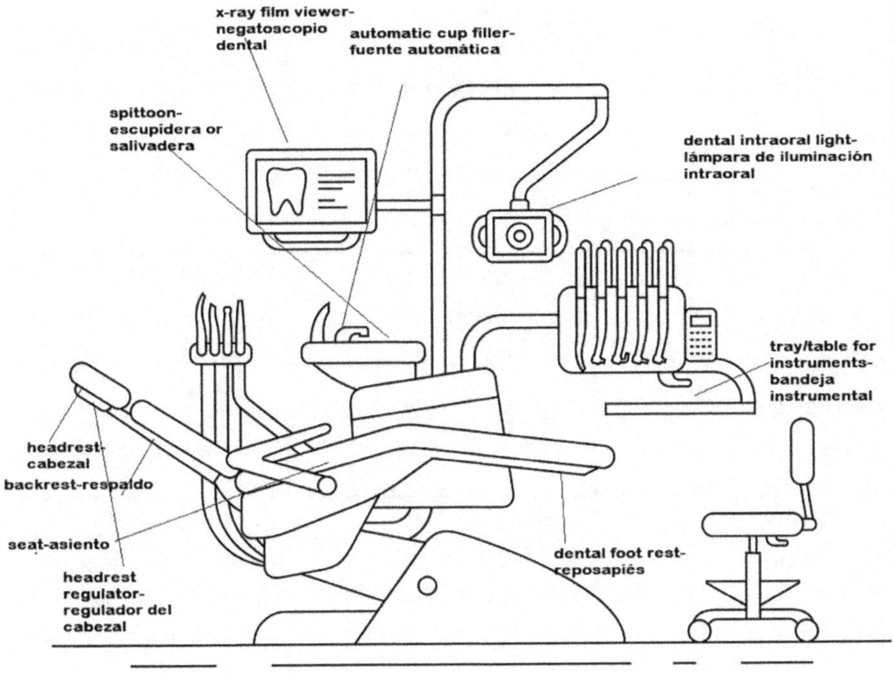
x-ray film viewer-
negatoscopio
dental
automatic cup filler-
fuente automática
spittoon-
escupidera or
salivadera
dental intraoral light-
lámpara de iluminación
intraoral
tray/table for
instruments-
bandeja
instrumental
headrest-
cabezal
backrest-respaldo
seat-asiento
headrest
regulator-
regulador del
cabezal
dental foot rest-
reposapiés

DENTAL TOOLS

 Dental drill or turbine → el taladro / la turbina dental	 Suction equipment → Equipo de succión Suction -el succionador	Dental tweezers → pinzas dentales
 Probes → las sondas Periodontal probe-sonda periodontal	Mouth mirror → el espejo dental or el espejo bucal 	Tongue depressor → depresor de lengua
 Dental plier → alicates dentales	Explorer → explorador dental 	Dental impression tray → cubeta para impresión
Dental excavator → excavadora dental 	Syringe → jeringa Air/Water Syringe-jeringa de aire/agua 	Dental scaler/ Ultrasonic scaler → escalador dental/ escalador ultrasónico
Dental extracting forceps → fórceps de extracción	Dental scalpel → bisturí dental 	Dental retractor → Retractor dental

Recepcionista/información preliminar del paciente, Receptionist/preliminary patient information

¿Cuál es su......?, What is your......?

> *nombre /apellido(nombre completo)?* name /last name (first and last name)?
> *sexo,* gender
> *dirección,* address
> *número de teléfono/celular,* home telephone number/cell number
> *fecha de nacimiento/lugar de nacimiento,* date of birth/place of birth
> *estatura/altura,* height
> *ocupación,* occupation
> *contacto en caso de emergencia,* emergency contact
> *lugar de trabajo,* place of work
> *grupo étnico, raza,* ethnic group
> *idioma primario,* primary language
> *número de seguro social,* social security number
> *tarjeta de seguro médico /de salud,* medical/health insurance card
> *tarjeta de medicaid (tarjeta de medicare),* medicaid card (medicare card)
> *¿Quién es el médico de su familia?* Who is your primary care physician or family doctor?

> *estado civil,* marital status
> *soltero/a,* single
> *casado/a,* married
> *separado/a,* separated
> *divorciado/a,* divorced
> *viudo/a,* widow/widower
> *unión civil,* domestic partnership

Direcciones al paciente, Directions to the patient

> Llene la planilla, por favor. Please fill out the form.
> *Espere un momento, por favor.* Wait one moment, please.
> *Enseguida le atiendo.* I will attend to you shortly.
> *Tome asiento, por favor or siéntese.* Take a seat, please.

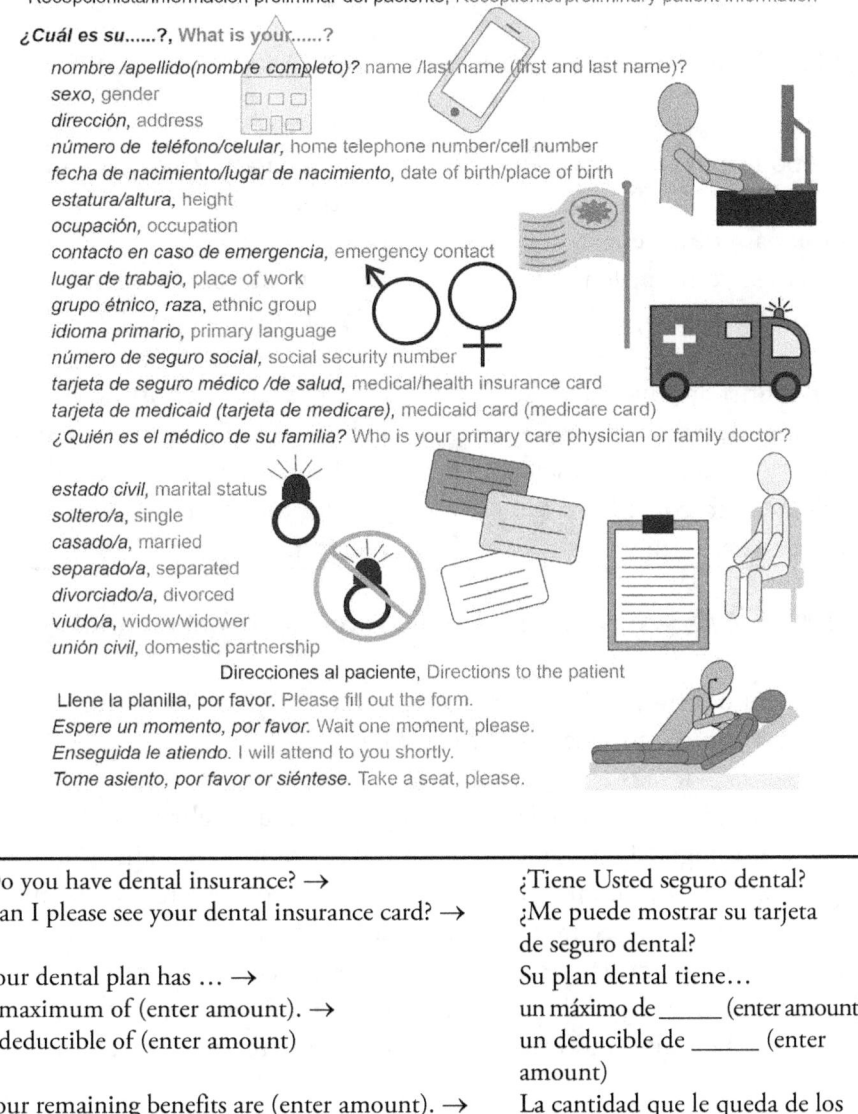

Do you have dental insurance? →	¿Tiene Usted seguro dental?
Can I please see your dental insurance card? →	¿Me puede mostrar su tarjeta de seguro dental?
Your dental plan has … →	Su plan dental tiene…
a maximum of (enter amount). →	un máximo de _____ (enter amount).
a deductible of (enter amount)	un deducible de _____ (enter amount)
Your remaining benefits are (enter amount). →	La cantidad que le queda de los beneficios es _____
Your dental plan covers (enter amount)% →	Su plan dental cubre (enter amount)%
Your covered services are … →	Sus servicios cubiertos son…
Your dental plan requires … →	Su plan dental requiere …
a referral for a specialist →	un referido para un especialista
advanced approval →	aprovación previa (autorización)
(an authorization) for certain procedures. →	para ciertos procedimientos.

DENTIST APPOINTMENTS	CITAS CON EL DENTISTA
You need……	Necesita……
an appointment with the dentist.	pedir una cita / hacer cita con el dentista
another appointment	otra cita
To change your appointment	cambiar su hora de la cita
To confirm your appointment	confirmar su cita
Your dentist appointment is…..	Su cita con el dentist está…….
on Monday, November 15th	el lunes, el quince de noviembre
Confirmed/cancelled/ rescheduled	confirmada/cancelada/cambiada
You'll need to come back for another appointment.	Tendrá que hacer otra cita para regresar.

CULTURA 🏁🏁🏁 National Dentist Day El día del odontólogo

El "Día del odontólogo" o "Día del dentista" (Day of the Dentist) is celebrated in various countries on different dates.

In Spain, México, Guatemala, Panamá y Nicaragua, February 9th is el Día de la Odontología. This coincides with the celebration of Saint Apollonia's Feast Day. Saint Apollonia was a devout Christian in the reign of Emperor Phillip who was persecuted for her religious beliefs. Part of her torture included pulling and shattering her teeth. Her teeth were broken one by one with rocks and scalding iron. Apollonia endured the torture without renouncing her faith and thus she became the patron saint of dentists.

October 3rd is el Día de la Odontología in Argentina, Bolivia, Colombia, Cuba, Ecuador, Paraguay, La República Dominicana, Uruguay and Venezuela. This coincides with the formation of the Latin American Dental Federation (FOLA), which was formed on October 3, 1917 in a Congress in Santiago de Chile.

March 6th is National Dentist's Day in the United States.

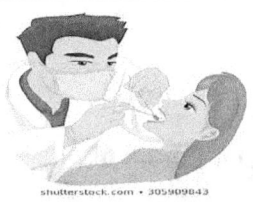

shutterstock.com · 305909843

DENTAL INITIAL CONSULTATION- CONSULTA DENTAL INICIAL

Hello, my name is Doctor_____.

Hola, soy el/la doctoro/doctora_____

When was your last dental appointment?

¿Cuándo fue su última cita / visita dental?

When was the last time you saw a dentist?

¿Cuándo fue la última vez que visitó al dentista?

Who was your last dentist?

¿Quién fue su previo dentista?

What is your chief complaint?

¿Cuál es su queja principal?

Are you having any dental problems?

¿Tiene algún problema dental?

How often do you brush your teeth?

¿Cuántas veces al día se cepilla los dientes?

Do your gums bleed?

¿Le sangran las encías?

Do you use dental floss?

¿Usa hilo dental?

Are you allergic to any medicines?

¿Es alérgico/alérgica a algún medicamento?

Are you allergic to antibiotics / penicillin?

¿Es alérgico a la penicilina/antibióticos?

I am going to take your vital signs.

Le voy a tomar sus signos vitales.

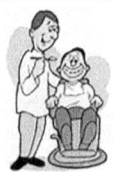

DENTAL EXAM   EXAMINACION DENTAL

Your tooth is…	Su diente está…
broken	roto
fractured	fracturado
infected	infectado
loose	flojo
I need an X-Ray of your tooth.	Necesito una radiografía de su diente.
I need to fix your broken tooth.	Tengo que reparar su diente roto.
I need to remove this tooth.	Tengo que sacarle este diente.
Your tooth is non-restorable.	Su diente no es restaurable.
You have _____cavities.	Tiene _____ caries.

OJO *take note* **IDIOMATIC EXPRESSIONS**. Idiomatic expressions are a type of informal language with a meaning that is different from the meaning of the words in the expression. In English, examples of idiomatic expressions are: It takes two to tango. Break a leg. Once in a blue moon. It's raining cats & dogs.

There are several idiomatic expressions in Spanish with the word **'diente'** that are unrelated with the anatomical part ('tooth'):

- darse con un canto en los dientes → to thank your lucky stars
- maldecir entre dientes → to curse under one's breath
- hablar entre dientes → to mumble; to speak under someone's breath
- enseñar los dientes → to threaten or to defend one's self; turn nasty
- poner los dientes largos a alguien → to make someone jealous
- decir algo para dientes afuera → to say one thing and mean another
- tener buen diente → to be a hearty eater
- estar a diente → to be ravenous

SPANISH PROVERB: *Más cerca están mis dientes que mis parientes. Charity begins at home.*

Collins Spanish Dictionary By HarperCollins Publishers. Available from: https://www.collinsdictionary.com › Browse the Spanish-English Dictionary. [Accessed 27 February 2023].

TYPES OF CAVITIES   LOS TIPOS DE CARIES

Cavity of the crown → carie de corona

Pit & Fissure cavity → carie de fosa y fisura

Recurring cavity → carie recurrente

Root cavity → carie radicular

Cavity between the teeth → carie interdental o interproximal

Cavity of the enamel → carie del esmalte

Signos vitales, Vital signs

Frecuencia respiratoria, Respiration rate

-disnea, dyspnea
-eupnea, eupnea
-bradipnea, bradypnea
-taquipnea, tachypnea
-apnea, apnea
-ortopenea, ortopnea
-hiperpnea, hyperpnea
-hiperventilación, hyperventilation
hipoventilación, hypoventilation

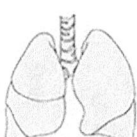

Pulso arterial y frecuencia cardiaca,
Pulse (heart rate) frecuencia cardiaca
(abbreviation: FC)

-los latidos cardíacos irregulares,
irregular heart beat
-bradicardia /bradisfignia, bradycardia
-taquicardia / taquisfignia, tachycardia
-pulso rápido/lento/ irregular/ normal,
fast/slow/irregular/normal pulse
-pulso hipocinético, hypokinetic pulse
-pulso hipercinético, hyperkinetic
pulse

La temperatura corporal, Body temperature
(abbreviation: TC)

-hipertermia, hyperthermia
-hipotermia, hypothermia

<u>Tipos de fiebre, Types of fever</u>

-febrícula, low grade fever
-fiebre moderada, moderate fever
-fiebre alta, high fever
-fiebre continua, continuous fever
-fiebre intermitente, intermittent fever
-fiebre recurrente, recurring fever
-fiebre ondulante, undulant fever

Tension arterial, Blood pressure
(abbreviation: TA)

-presión baja/la presión alta, low blood pressure/
high blood pressure
-hipertensión/hipotensión, hypertension/
hypotension
-presión normal/alta/baja, normal/high/low blood
pressure
-la presión sistólica, systolic pressure
-la presión diastólica, diastolic pressure

VITAL SIGN- SIGNO VITAL	REQUESTING PERMISSION / GIVING INSTRUCTIONS TO THE PATIENT-PEDIR PERMISO/DAR INSTRUCCIONES AL PACIENTE	GIVING RESULTS TO THE PATIENT DAR RESULTADOS AL PACIENTE
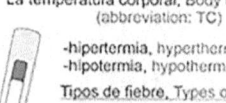 The pulse-el pulso	Can I take your pulse? ¿Me permite tomar su pulso?	You have a fast/slow/ normal/irregular/pulse. Su pulso es rápido/lento/ normal/irregular. Your pulse is __per minute. Su pulso está en __ por minute.

  Heart beat-latidos cardíacos	 Can I check your heart rate? ¿Me permite comprobar su ritmo cardíaco?	 Your heart beat is irregular/fast/slow. Sus latidos cardíacos son irregulares/rápidos/lentos
  The oxygen-el oxígeno	 Can I measure your oxygen level? ¿Me permite medirle el oxígeno?	 Your oxygen is 98%. Su oxigeno está en 98% (por ciento)
  Blood pressure-la presión arterial	 Can I please take your blood pressure? ¿Me permite tomar su presión arterial?	 You have high / low blood pressure. Usted tiene presión arterial alta/ baja.
  Temperature-temperatura	 Can I take your temperature? ¿Me permite tomarle la temperatura	 You have a low grade fever. Tiene febricula. You have a moderate/high/continuous/intermittent fever. Tiene una fiebre moderada/alta/continua/intermitente.

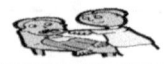
Abscess tooth → diente con absceso	Baby cavities → caries de biberón Baby teeth → Dientes de leche	Bad breath → Mal aliento/ la halitosis	Bleeding/ hemorrhage → sangrado/ hemorragia	Blister → una ampolla	Broken teeth → dientes quebrados/ rotos Broken fillings → Rellenos quebrados
Canker sore → úlcera de la boca/úlcera aftosa/afta	Cavities → caries	Clicking or popping jaw → ruido en la quijada	Cracked tooth → diente roto / diente quebrado	Crooked teeth → dientes torcidos Crooked bite-mordida torcida	Decay → desgaste Decayed tooth-diente deteriorado
Dry mouth → boca seca	Enamel loss → pérdida de esmalte	Food collection between teeth → Se junta comida entre los dientes	Gingival swelling → inflamación de las encías Gingivitis-gingivitis	Grinding teeth → rechina de los dientes	Gum bleeding → Sangrado de las encías

12

Gum inflammation → inflamación	Hyperdontia→ hiperdoncia	Impacted tooth → diente traumatizado Impacted wisdom teeth → muelas de juicio impactadas	Infected tooth → diente infectado	Loose teeth → dientes flojos	Lump → masa
Missing teeth → dientes que faltan	Mouth sores or growths → bultos o llagas cerca de su boca	Mouth wounds or irritations → llagas bucales o irritaciones	Occlusion → oclusión Malocclusion-maloclusión	Oral cancer → cáncer oral	Plaque → placa
Sensitive gums → encías sensibles	Sensitive teeth → dientes sensibles	Sensitivity to hot → sensible a lo caliente	Sensitivity to sweets → sensible a lo dulce	Sensitivity to cold → sensible a lo frio	Sensitive to biting → sensible cuando muerde
Stained teeth → dientes manchados	Swelling → hinchazón	Toothache → dolor de muelas	Ulcers (mouth) → úlceras bucales	Warts (mouth) → verrugas de la boca	Wisdom tooth pain → dolor de muelas de juicio

Terminología dental común, Common dental terminology

diente con absceso, abscess tooth

diente de leche, baby tooth

blanqueamiento, bleaching

los frenos para los dientes; los frenillos para los dientes, braces

afta, canker sore

caries, cavities

diente roto/diente quebrado, cracked tooth

dientes torcidos, crooked tooth

desgaste, decay

obturaciones, empastes, dental filling

hilo dental, dental floss

FLOSS

la higiene bucal, dental hygiene

dentadura postiza, denture

boca seca, dry mouth

exodoncia, extraction
sacar una muela, extract a tooth

diente extruído, extruding tooth
diente intruído, intruding tooth

flúor-florización, fluoride

hacer gárgaras, to gargle

halitosis, el mal aliento crónico, halitosis

diente traumatizado, impacted tooth

implante, implant

diente infectado, infected tooth

diente flojo, loose tooth

dientes que faltan, missing teeth

enjuague bucal, mouth wash

ortodoncia, orthodontics

periodoncia, periodontics/
periodontitis, periodontitis

placa, plaque

el retenedor, retainer

endodoncia, root canal

dientes sensibles, sensitive teeth
/encías sensibles, sensitive gums

hinchazón, swelling

cepillarse los dientes, to brush one's teeth

dolor de muelas, tooth ache

limpieza dental, tooth cleaning

Dental Hygiene-La higiene dental

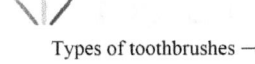

Types of toothbrushes → 　　　　　　　　Types of bristles → Tipos de cerdas
Tipos de cepillos de dientes

Conventional tooth brush → el cepillo convencional Electric toothbrush → el cepillo eléctrico Periodontal tooth brush → el cepillo periodontal Interproximal tooth brush → el cepillo interproximal Sonic toothbrush → el cepillo sónico	Hard → duros Medium → medios Soft → suaves Extra-soft → extra suaves

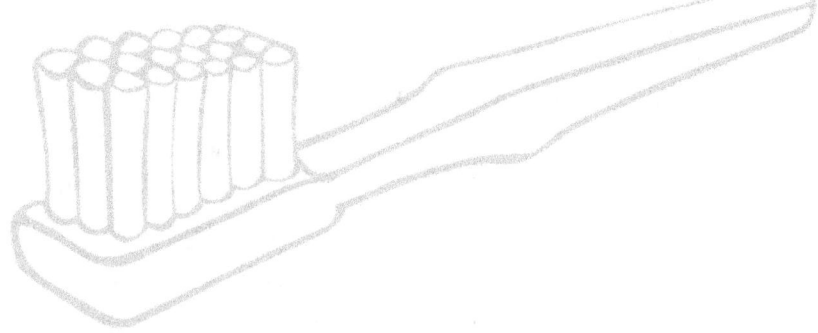

Types of toothpastes 　　　　　　　　**Tipos de pasta de dientes**
Anti-cavity → Pasta dental anticaries
Anti-plaque toothpaste → Pasta dental antiplaca
Fluoride toothpaste→ pasta dental con flúor
Fluoride-free toothpaste→ pasta dental libre de flúor
Organic toothpastes→ pasta dental orgánica
Periodontal disease tooth paste → Pasta de dientes para enfermedades periodontales
Sensitive Gum tooth paste → Pasta de dientes para encías sensibles
Sensitive teeth tooth paste → Pasta de dientes para dientes sensibles/ para la sensibilidad dentaria
Tartar-control tooth paste → pasta dental antisarro
Whitening toothpaste → Pasta dental blanqueadora

15

ORAL HYGIENE TERMINOLOGY VOCABULARIO PARA LA HIGIENE BUCAL

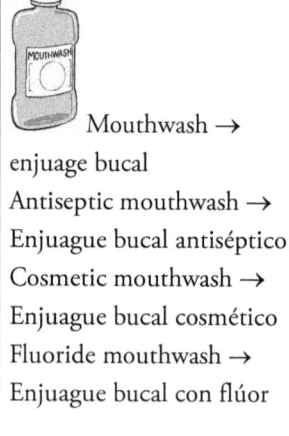 Mouthwash → enjuage bucal Antiseptic mouthwash → Enjuague bucal antiséptico Cosmetic mouthwash → Enjuague bucal cosmético Fluoride mouthwash → Enjuague bucal con flúor	Dental floss → el hijo dental Biodegradable floss → El hilo dental biodegradable Flavored and unflavored floss → hilo dental con sabor/sin sabor Tape floss / dental tape → cinta dental Waxed and unwaxed floss → hilo dental con cera/sin cera	Fluoride → flúor/florización Toothpaste with fluoride → pasta de dientes con flúor Fluoride gel → gel con flúor Dental varnishes with fluoride → barnices para dientes con flúor Mouthwash with fluoride → enjuague con flúor Dental Floss with fluoride → seda dental fluorada

Tooth Brushing Techniques Terms→ 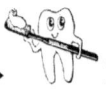 **La técnica de cepillado**

Cleaning of the chewing areas → Limpieza de las zonas masticatorias

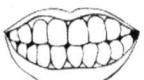

Tongue cleaning → Limpieza de la lengua

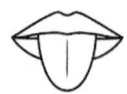

Cleaning of the internal surfaces of the teeth → Limpieza de las superficies internas.

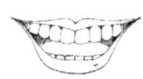

Cleaning of the exernal surfaces of the teeth. → Limpieza de las superficies externas.

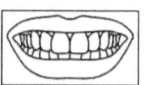

TOOTH BRUSHING

Do you brush your teeth daily?

Do you brush your teeth after eating?

Do you brush your teeth at night before sleeping?

CEPILLARSE LOS DIENTES

¿Se cepilla los dientes diariamente?/ todos los días?

¿Se cepilla los dientes después de comer?

¿Se cepilla los dientes por la noche antes de dormir?

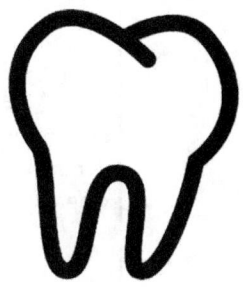

How many times a day do you brush your teeth?
Do you / does he/she use...
dental floss?

¿Cuántas veces al día se cepilla los dientes?
¿Usa...?
hilo dental?

Tooth scaling→ raspado/raspar los dientes	Tooth cleaning→ limpiar los dientes	Tooth polishing→ pulir los dientes
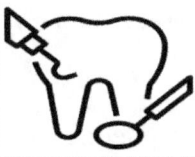	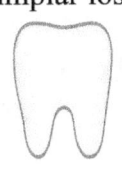	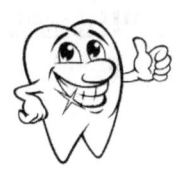

Are your teeth sensitive to...
scaling
cleaning
I am going to...
clean your teeth.
polish your teeth.
scale your teeth

¿Son sensibles sus dientes ...
al raspado?
a la limpieza?
Le voy a...
limpiar sus dientes.
pulir los dientes.
raspar los dientes.

17

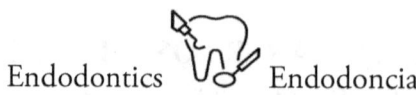

Endodontics   Endodoncia

<u>Root Canal Vocabulary-El conducto radicular</u>

Tooth /pulp infection → Infección del diente/ de la pulpa Dental abscess → absceso dental	Cleaning of root canal → limpieza de los conductos radiculares Filing & scraping of root canal → raspar y limar los conductos radiculares	Filling of the root canal → relleno del conducto radicular Dental filling → obturación, empaste Temporary filling → empaste provisional	Temporary or permanent crown → una corona temporal/ permanente

ENDODONTIC TOOLS

Endodontic file → la lima de endodoncia	Rubber dam → el dique de goma	Sealant → sellado radicular

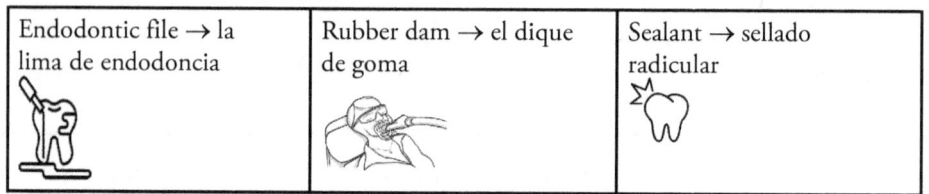

<u>USEFUL PHRASES</u>

The root of the tooth is fine.

La raíz del diente aparece bien en la radiografía.

This tooth can/ can not be saved.

Este diente puede / no puede ser salvado.

You need a root canal.

Necesita un conducto radicular.

After the root canal, you will need a crown.

Después de completar el canal radicular, necesitará una corona.

Orthodontics-Ortodoncia para los dientes

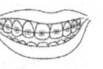

Braces-los frenos/ los frenillos

BRACES & THEIR PARTS

LOS FRENILLOS Y SUS PARTES

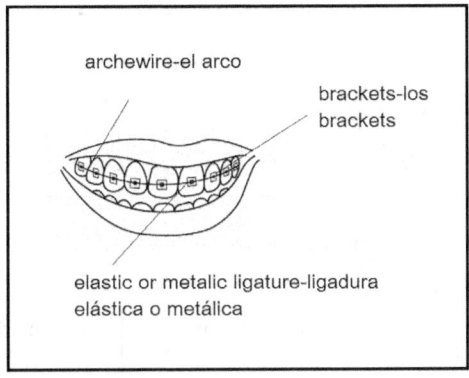

archewire-el arco

brackets-los brackets

elastic or metalic ligature-ligadura elástica o metálica

Types of Braces → tipos de frenos/frenillos

metal → frenillos metálicos
ceramic → frenillos de cerámica
lingual → frenillos linguales
clear aligners → los alineadores transparentes

Orthodontic Issues

Widely spaced teeth → dientes muy espaciados / separación entre los dientes	Overbite → sobremordida	Crowded teeth → apiñamiento	Crooked teeth→ dientes torcidos
Open bite → Mordida abierta	Cross bite → Mordida cruzada	Underbite → submordida	Occlusion / Malocclusion → oclusión/ maloclusión

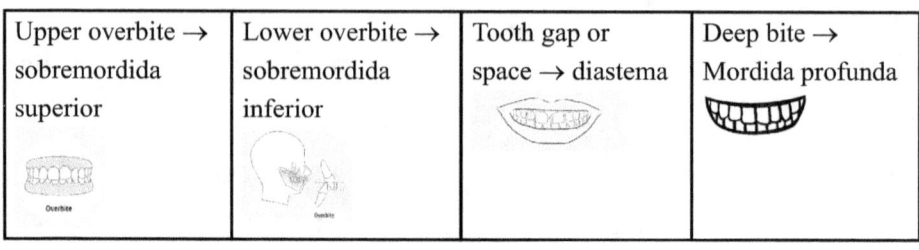

Upper overbite → sobremordida superior	Lower overbite → sobremordida inferior	Tooth gap or space → diastema	Deep bite → Mordida profunda

Periodontics  **Periodoncia**

PERIODONTAL AILMENTS

Bleeding gums when grushing or flossing → sangrado de las encías al cepillarse los dientes o al usar hilo dental	Red, swollen, tender gums → encias rojas e hinchadas	Chronic bad breath (Halitosis) → mal aliento crónico	Hot and/or cold sensitive teeth → dientes sensibles al calor/al frío	Loose teeth (in adults) → dientes sueltos (en adultos)
Gum recession → una recesión de las encías / encías que retroceden	Pain when chewing → dolor al masticar	Gum disease → enfermedad de las encías	Plaque → placa	Tartar removal → tartrectomía

Periodontitis Treatment
Gum Grafts → injerto de encía quirúrgico
Bone Grafting → injertos óseos
Scaling and Root Planing → raspado y alisado radicular
Periodontal surgery → Cirugía periodontal
Periodontal regeneration → Regeneración periodontal

Prosthodontics – Prostodoncia

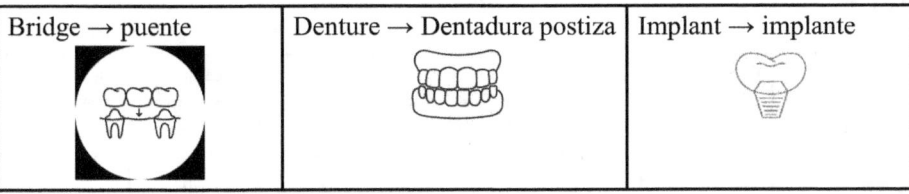

Bridge → puente	Denture → Dentadura postiza	Implant → implante

Types of Implants  **Tipos de implantes dentales**

Endosteal Implants → Endo-áseos
Subperiosteal Implants → Subperióticos
Zygomatic → zigomáticos
Pterygoid implants- Pterigoideos
Implant Overdentures → sobredentaduras soportadas por implantes

Types of Dentures 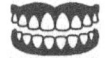 **Tipos de dentaduras postizas:**

- Acrylic dentures → dentadura postiza fija acrílica
- Custom dentures → dentaduras postizas personalizadas
- Full dentures → dentadura completa removible
- Hybrid Dentures → dentadura postiza fija híbrida
- Implant-supported fixed dentures → dentadura fija sobre implantes
- Overdentures → sobredentaduras postizas
- Partial dentures → dentaduras parciales
- Temporary dentures → dentaduras postizas temporalis
- Upper dentures → dentaduras superiores

Types of crowns Tipos de coronas

Gold crown → corona dental de aleación de oro	Ceramic crown → corona dental de cerámica	Porcelain crown → corona de porcelana	Ceramic crown over metal → corona de cerámica sobre metal	Metal crown → corona de metal	Porcelain fused to metal crown → corona de porcelana fusionada con metal	Zirconia crown → corona de zirconio

Cosmetic Dentistry   Estética dental

Tooth whitening → blanqueamiento dental	Cosmetic dental implants → implantes dentarios cosméticos	Dental veneers → carillasdentales	Cosmetic dental crowns → coronas dentales cosméticas	Cosmetic dental molds → modelado cosmético de dientes
Enamel decay → abrasión del esmalte	Cosmetic or adult orthodontia → ortodoncia cosmética	Cosmetic Bridges → puentes cosméticos	Dentures → dentaduras postizas	Remodeling and grafting of the gum → remodelado e injerto de encía

DENTAL SEDATION & ANESTHESIA VOCABULARY   TIPOS DE SEDACION DENTAL Y ANESTESIA

Local anesthetic → anesthesia local	General anesthetic → Anestesia general	Sedation → Sedación	Analgesic → analgésico
Topical Anesthesia → La anesthesia tópica Anesthetic spray, cream, patch or gel → Espray, crema, parche o gel anestésico	Intravenous (IV) sedation → sedación intravenosa	Nitrous oxide (laughing gas) → El óxido nitroso (gas de la risa) Sleepy Juice → el jugo para dormir	

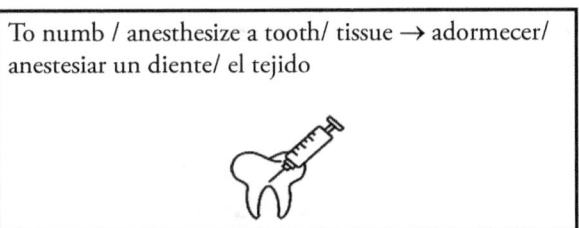

To numb / anesthesize a tooth/ tissue → adormecer/ anestesiar un diente/ el tejido

ANESTHESIA

Have you ever had an allergic reaction to anesthesia?

I will numb your tooth.

I will place gel in the interior of your mouth to numb the tissue.

You will feel a sting from the anesthesia.

Tell me if your lip (face) feel numb.

ANESTESIA

¿Alguna vez ha tenido una reacción alérgica a la anestesia?

Voy a adormecer su diente.

Colocaré gel en el interior de su boca para adormecer el tejido.

Va a sentir una picadura de la anestesia.

Dígame si su labio (cara) se siente adormecido.

Radiographic Examination

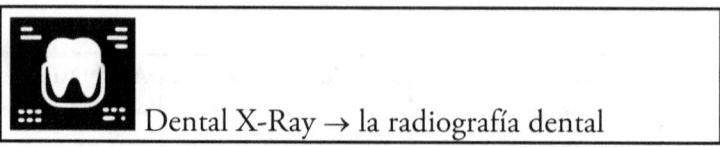

Dental X-Ray → la radiografía dental

Equipment for Dental X-Rays   Equipo para radiografías dentales

Dental chair → silla dental	Lead apron → delantal de plomo	Thyroid collar → el collar de tiroides	Sensor or X-Ray film → el sensor o la película de rayos X	X-Ray machine → la máquina de rayos or de radiografías

USEFUL X-RAY PHRASES

I need to take an X-Ray for this tooth.	Necesito tomar una radiografía de este diente.
Do you have previous dental x-rays?	¿Tiene radiografías de su previo dentist?
May I contact your previous dentist for dental x-rays?	¿Me permite contactar a su dentista previo para radiografías?
The machine will rotate around you for __ seconds.	La máquina rotará alrederdor de Usted por _____segundos

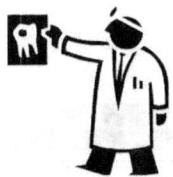

Dental X-Ray Vocabulary Rayos X Dentales

- Bitewing X-Ray → la radiografía de tipo bitewing or la radiografía interproximal, aleta de mórdida
- Cephalometric Projection → Cefalometría
- Cone Beam X-ray → Tomografía computarizada (TC) dental de haz cónico
- Dental C.A.T. (Computed Axial Tomography) → TAC Dental
- Orthopantomography → Ortopantomografía
- Occlusal X-Ray → la radiografía occlusal
- Panoramic X-Ray → la radiografía panorámica
- Periapical X-Ray → la radiografía periapical

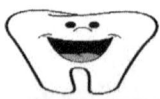

SAMPLE DENTAL INTAKE FORM

Patient Information: Información del paciente:

Name of the patient: Nombre del paciente:
Date of Birth:_ _ / _ /__ _ Fecha de nacimiento:_ _ / _ /__ _
Address: City, State, Zip Code Dirección: Cuidad, Estado, Código Postal:
Social Security Number: Número de seguro social: _____
Home Telephone Number:_____ Número de teléfono de Casa: Cell Number:_____ ( )- - Número de celular: ( )- - _____ Work Telephone Number: Número de trabajo: ( )- - _____ E-Mail Address: Correo electrónico:
Referred by: Referido por:

Emergency Contact Information   **Información de contacto en caso de emergencia**

Name of the emergency contact: Nombre del contacto de emergencia:
Relationship to the patient: Relación con el paciente:
Home Telephone Teléfono de casa: Cell telephone number: Número de celular

DENTAL HISTORY_____   HISTORIA DENTAL
Reason for today's visit:_____ Razón por la que vino hoy: _____
Date of last dental visit_____ Fecha de su última visita al dentista_____
Dentist Name:_____ Nombre del dentista_____

Check if you have had problems with any of the following: Marque si ha tenido algún problema de los siguientes:

_____Bad Breath _____ Mal aliento ___	___ Grinding teeth ___ Rechina los dientes ___
___ Bleeding gums _____ Sangrado de encía	___ Loose teeth _____ Dientes flojos _____
___ Broken fillings _____ Rellenos quebrados	___Sensitivity to hot /cold/sweets/biting- Sensible a lo caliente / frío / a lo dulce/ cuando muerde
___ Clicking or popping jaw ___ Ruido en la quijada	_____ Sores or growths in your mouth _____ Bultos o llagas cerca de su boca
_____ Food collection between teeth _____ Se junta comida entre los dientes	___Use of dentures (partial) ___usa dentaduras postizas o parciales

DENTAL HYGIENE HABITS   HIGIENE ORAL

How often do you brush?_____	¿Cada cuando se cepilla?_____
How often do you floss?_____	¿ Cada cuando usa el hilo dental?_____

MEDICAL HISTORY   HISTORIA MEDICA

Physician's Name:_____ Nombre de su doctor:_____

Date of last visit:_____ Fecha de su última visita:_____

Have you had any serious illnesses or operations? ___ ¿ Ha tenido alguna operación o enfermedad grave?___

Describe_____ Explique_____

List medications you are currently taking   Anote cualquier medicamento que este tomando

Check here if none □ Marque aquí si ninguno □

Name of the Medication Nombre de la medicación	Dosage dosis	Frequency Frecuencia

Are you allergic to any medication? ¿ Es alérgico,a a algún medicamento?_____

(Women) ___(Mujeres)

Are you pregnant? __Yes __No Embaraza?__Sí__No
Nursing?__Yes __No Amamantando?__Sí__No
Taking birth control pills? __Yes __No ¿Toma pastillas anticonceptivas?__Sí__No

Check if you have or have had any of the following: Marque si tiene o ha tenido algo de lo siguiente:

___Anemia ___anemia	□	___Hepatitis ___Hepatitis	□
___Arthritis___artritis	□	___High Blood Pressure _____ Alta Presión	□
___Artificial Heart Valves __Válvulas artificiales del corazón	□	___HIV/AIDS _____Sida o HIV	□
___Asthma __asma	□	___Kidney Disease___Enfermedad de riñon	□
___Back Problems Problemas de espalda	□	___Liver Disease___Enfermedad de hígado	□
___Blood Disease Enfermedad de la sangre	□	___Pacemaker_____ Marcapasos	□
___Cancer ___cáncer	□	___Radiation Treatment _____ Tratamiento de radiación	□
___Circulatory problems __ problemas circulatorios	□	___Respiratory Illnesses_____ Problemas respiratorios	□
___Cough, Persistent ___Tos persistente	□	___Shortness of Breath ___Falta de aliento	□
___Diabetes _____diabetes	□	___Stroke _____derrame cerebral	□
___Epilepsy ___Epilepsia	□	___Thyroid Problems ___ ___Problema de tiroides	□
___Fainting___Desmayos	□	___Ulcers ___Ulceras	□
___Heart Problems/Murmur ___ Problemas del corazón/soplo cardíaco	□	___Venereal Disease___Enfermedad venérea	□

PAIN   EL DOLOR

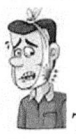

THE NOUN- EL DOLOR –THE PAIN

The noun 'dolor' means 'pain'. One way to express pain is to use the verb *'tener'*. Use the construction ***tener dolor de + body part*/tooth.** This literally means : To have pain of + body part/tooth . Example : Tengo dolor de la muela. My tooth hurts. Literally : I have pain of the tooth.

OJO *take note* The verb tener-to have- is an irregular verb.

The following are the conjugations: yo tengo, tú tienes, él, ella, Usted tiene, nosotros tenemos, vosotros tenéis, ellos, Ustedes tienen.
Example: Juan has a a toothache. Juan tiene dolor de las muelas.

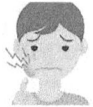

OJO *take note* **You do not use a possessive to refer to the body part.**

You use the indefinite article (el,la, los, las).
THE VERB DOLER-TO HURT

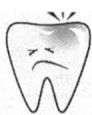

The verb ***doler*** is an o: ue stem changing verb. The two most commonly used forms are the third person singular ***duele*** or the third person plural ***duelen.*** The doler construction is similar to the gustar construction. The subject is the part or parts of the body that hurt. In Spanish , the literal translation of doler + body part is that the body part hurts.

In English we say: My gums hurt. In Spanish we say: Me duelen las encías. Literally: The gums hurt me. The indirect object pronoun is placed before ***duele / duelen*** and expresses the recipient of the pain.

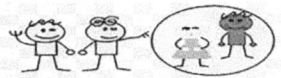

INDIRECT OBJECT PRONOUN-IDOP-Whom does it hurt
Me -to me
Te -to you (familiar)
Le- to him, to her or to you (formal)
Nos -to us
Os -to you all (used in Spain)
Les to them, or to you all (Latin America)

OJO *take note* The third person IDOP, ***le*** can mean 'to him' , 'to her' , 'to you (formal)', to it (such as a pet). To determine which person it is referring to, use context (what came before) or a clarifier. Example- Le duele el diente **a Juan**. Juan's tooth hurts. The third person plural IDOP, ***les,*** can mean 'to them' or 'to you (all)'. Meaning is determined by context (what came before) or a clarifier. Example: Les duele el diente **a Juan y Julia**. Their (Juan's & Julia's tooth hurts).

DOLER –TO HURT
3- PART CONSTRUCTION

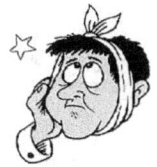

IDOP + duele IF ONE BODY PART / ONE TOOTH/ONE MOUTH PART OR JAW HURTS
IDOP + duelen IF MORE THAN ONE BODY PART / MORE THAN ONE TOOTH HURT

OJO *take note* **You do not use a possessive to refer to the body part. You use the indefinite article (el,la, los, las). The recipient of pain is expressed in the IDOP (Indirect Object Pronoun).**

Me duele la muela/ el diente. My tooth hurts.
(LITERAL: The tooth hurts me).

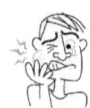

Your (familiar) jaw hurts. Te duele la mandíbula.
(LITERAL: The jaw hurts you (familiar).

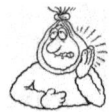

His/her/ your(formal) gums hurt. Le duelen las encías.
(LITERAL: The gums hurt you (formal) /him/her).

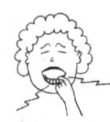

Our teeth hurt. Nos duelen las muelas/los dientes.
(LITERAL: Our teeth hurt us).

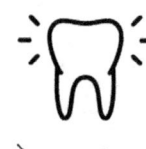

Your (all-Spain) gums hurt. Os duelen las encías.
(LITERAL: The gums hurt to you all).

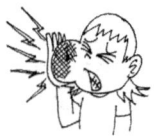

Their/ your (all-Latin America) mouth hurts.
Les duele la boca. (LITERAL: The mouth hurts you all or them).

DENTIST PAIN ASSESSMENT 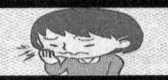 -EL DOLOR

PAIN HISTORY

How long ago did the pain start?	¿Hace cuánto empezó el dolor?
How did your tooth get hurt?	¿Cómo se lastimó el diente?

GENERAL PAIN QUESTIONS

Does it hurt?	¿Le duele?
Do you feel any pain in your mouth?	¿Ud. siente algun tipo de dolor en su boca?
Can you point to the area that hurts?	¿Puede apuntar a la zona que le duele?
Does it hurt when you bite?	¿Le duele cuando muerde?
Does it hurt when I touch the tooth?	¿Le duele cuando toco el diente?
Does it hurt when I press here?	¿Le duele cuando aprieto aquí?
Does it hurt when you open & close your mouth?	¿Le duele cuando abre y cierra la boca?
Does the cold water or air hurt you?	¿Le molesta el agua o el aire frío?
Does anything make the pain worse?	¿Hay algo que empeora el dolor?
Describe the pain from a scale of 1-10, with 1 being the least painful	Describe el dolor en la escala del 1-10, con el 1 siendo el nivel más bajo del dolor

PAIN DURATION

How long has it hurt?	¿Por cuánto tiempo le ha dolido?
When does it hurt?	¿Cuándo le duele?

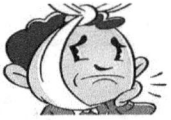

PAIN LOCATION

Where does it hurt?	¿Dónde le duele?
Point to where it hurts	Señale al lugar del dolor.
Where does it hurt the most?	¿Dónde más le duele?
Can you please show me where it hurts?	¿Me puede señalar donde le duele?

GENERAL PAIN EXPRESSIONS

It doesn't hurt. No me duele.	It hurts a little. Me duele un poquito.	The pain is unbearable. El dolor es insoportable.	The pain is sharp. El dolor es agudo.	The pain is dull. El dolor es sordo.
The pain is chronic. El dolor es crónico.	The pain is intense. El dolor es intenso.	I have pain that lasts a short duration. Tengo dolor de corta dura-ción.	I have long term pain. Tengo dolor que dura mucho. tiempo.	It hurts a lot. Me duele mucho.
It is pain with pressure. Es dolor con presión.	It is intermittent pain that comes and goes. Es dolor que va y viene (dolor intermitente).	The pain is constant. El dolor es constante.	The pain is throbbing. El dolor es punzante.	The pain is sharp and fleeting. El dolor es agudo y fugaz.

TYPES OF TOOTH PAIN -TIPOS DE DOLORES DENTALES

I feel pain with cold food/drinks. Siento dolor de dientes con el frío.	My tooth hurts when I bite. Me duele la muela/el diente al morder.	My tooth hurts when I touch it. Me duele la muela/ el diente al tocarlo.	I have sharp tooth pain/ sensitivity Tengo dolor den-tal agudo / o sen-sibilidad aguda.	I have tooth pain when I eat. Tengo dolor al comer.
I feel pain with hot food/drinks. Siento dolor de dientes con el el calor.	Water bothers me. Me molesta el agua.	Cold air bothers my tooth. Me molesta el aire frío.	My tooth hurts when I chew. Me duele la muela/el diente al masticar.	My teeth hurt when I eat something sweet. Me duelen los dientes al comer cosas con azúcar.

INSTRUCTIONS TO PATIENT ▲ INSTRUCCIONES AL PACIENTE

INSTRUCTIONS BEFORE DENTAL APPOINTMENT

Relax.	í Relájese!
Remain calm.	í Manténgase calmado!
Remove your lipstick..jewelery.	í Quítese su lápiz labial..joyas, por favor!
Speak slower, please.	í Hable más despacio, por favor!

INSTRUCTIONS DURING DENTAL APPOINTMENT

Bite slowly /bite again.
í Muerda despacio! / í Muerda otra vez!

Breathe through your nose.	í Respire por la naríz!
Close your mouth, please.	í Cierre la boca, por favor!
Hold still.	í No se mueva!
Lower/raise your chin.	í Baje/suba el mentón / la barbilla!
Open your mouth, please.	í Abra la boca, por favor.
Open wide/wider.	í Abra grande/ más grande!
Place your tongue on the roof of your mouth.	í Coloque su lengua contra el paladar!
Rinse, please.	í Enjuágese , por favor!
Spit out, please.	í Escupa, por favor!
Stick out your tongue.	í Saque la lengua, por favor!
Tap your teeth together, please.	í Choque sus dientes unos con otros!
Touch the root of your mouth with your tongue.	í Toque el techo de su boca con su lengua!
Turn your head to the right /left.	í Voltee la cabeza a la derecha/ a la izquierda!

INSTRUCTIONS AFTER DENTAL APPOINTMENT

Call me if it does not get better.	Llámeme si no mejora.
Do not eat or drink for _____minutes/hours.	No coma ni beba por _____ minutos/horas.
Do not chew on this side for _____minutes/hours.	No mastique en este lado por _____minutos/horas.
Do not brush tonight.	No se cepille esta noche.

ANATOMY

La cabeza, The head

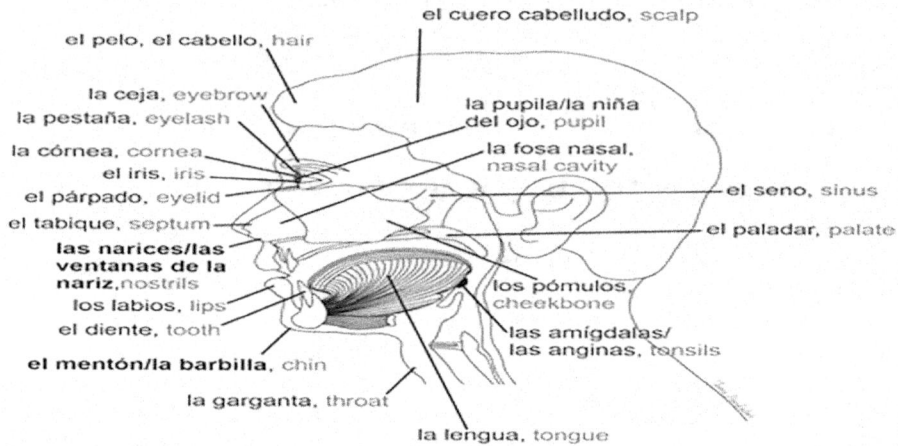

el cuero cabelludo, scalp

el pelo, el cabello, hair

la ceja, eyebrow

la pestaña, eyelash

la córnea, cornea

el iris, iris

el párpado, eyelid

el tabique, septum

las narices/las ventanas de la nariz, nostrils

los labios, lips

el diente, tooth

el mentón/la barbilla, chin

la garganta, throat

la pupila/la niña del ojo, pupil

la fosa nasal, nasal cavity

el seno, sinus

el paladar, palate

los pómulos, cheekbone

las amígdalas/las anginas, tonsils

la lengua, tongue

Boca, Mouth

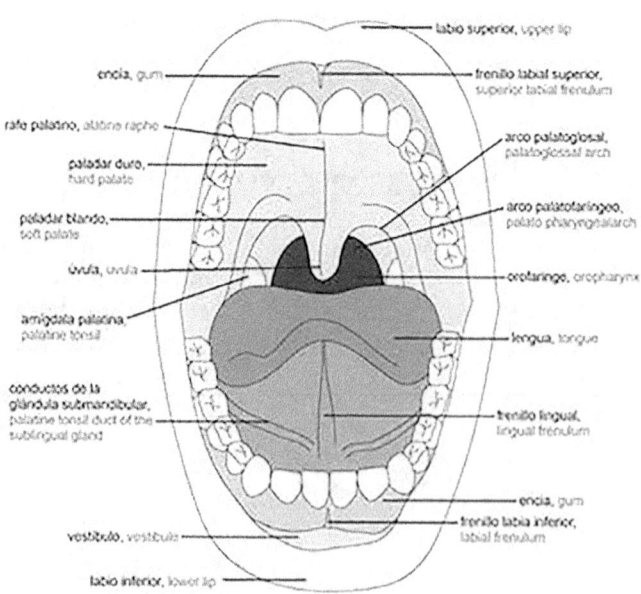

labio superior, upper lip

encía, gum

rafe palatino, palatine raphe

paladar duro, hard palate

paladar blando, soft palate

úvula, uvula

amígdala palatina, palatine tonsil

conductos de la glándula submandibular, palatine tonsil duct of the sublingual gland

vestíbulo, vestibule

labio inferior, lower lip

frenillo labial superior, superior labial frenulum

arco palatoglosal, palatoglossal arch

arco palatofaríngeo, palato pharyngeal arch

orofaringe, oropharynx

lengua, tongue

frenillo lingual, lingual frenulum

encía, gum

frenillo labia inferior, labial frenulum

34

Anatomía del diente, Tooth anatomy

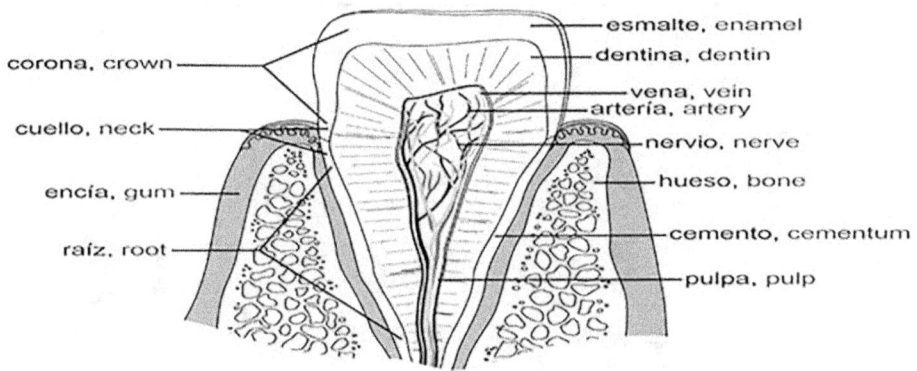

corona, crown

cuello, neck

encía, gum

raíz, root

esmalte, enamel

dentina, dentin

vena, vein
artería, artery

nervio, nerve

hueso, bone

cemento, cementum

pulpa, pulp

Los dientes, The teeth

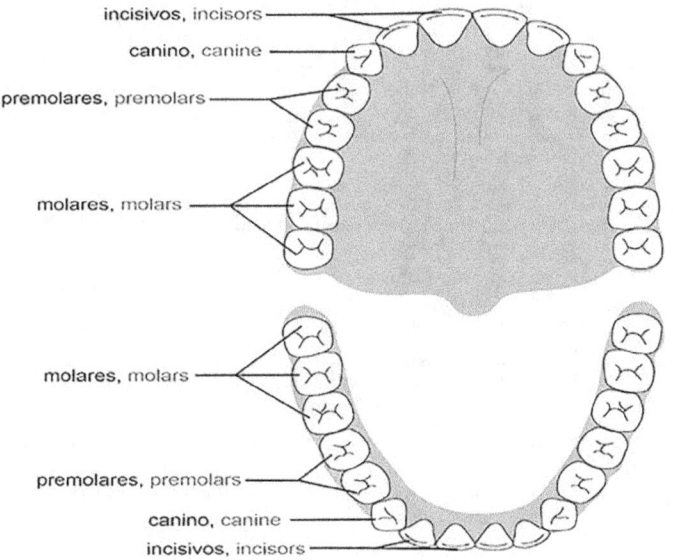

incisivos, incisors

canino, canine

premolares, premolars

molares, molars

molares, molars

premolares, premolars

canino, canine

incisivos, incisors

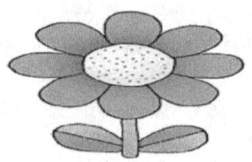

BASIC EXPRESSIONS   & GRAMMAR

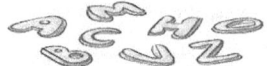

Alfabeto

Alphabet in Spanish, El Abecedario (Alfabeto)

Letter	Letter Name	Pronunciation	Example
A	a	Sounds like the English *ah*	ambulancia
B	be (also called be larga, be grande or be de burro)	Often sounds like the English *b*. When between 2 vowels, it is pronounced much like the Spanish *v* (lips not touching)	biopsia
C	ce	Sounds like an English *s* if followed by a soft vowel (e or i). Sounds like an English *k*, if followed by a consonant or a hard vowel (a, o, u)	cirugía camilla
CH	che	Sounds like an English *ch*; no longer considered a letter by RAE	chata
D	de	Sounds much like the English *d*. It is usually a softer sound, like *th* in English, especially when between 2 vowels	doctor
E	e	Sounds like *eh* in English	emergencia
F	efe	Sounds like an English *f*	fiebre (106°)
G	ge	Sounds like an English *g*, if followed by a consonant or a hard vowel (a, o,u); sounds like a harsh h if followed by a soft vowel (e or i).	ginecólogo gaza
H	hache	As a general rule, this letter is silent if it is the first letter of a word. The exception to this rule are words adopted from other languages, which maintain the breathy aspiration, such as Hawáii.	hospital
I	i	Sounds like *ee* in English, but shorter	insulina
J	jota	Sounds like *h* in English	jeringa
K	ca	Sounds like *k* in English. The letter K is not native to the Spanish language & only appears in loanwords such as karate, kilo	kilómetro
L	ele	Sounds like the English *l*, (tongue raised closer to the roof of the mouth; not dipped)	laringitis
LL	doble ele	Sounds like 'y' in English (no longer considered a letter by RAE)	llaga

36

M	eme	Sounds like the English *m*	mamografía
N	ene	Sounds like the English *n*	neurología
Ñ	eñe	Sounds like the *ni in onion* or the *ny* in *canyon*	riñon
O	o	Sounds like the *o* in *so*, but shorter	operación
P	pe	Sounds like an English *p*	paperas
Q	cu	Always followed by a *u* and sounds like the English *k*	quemadura
R	erre	Sounds like the English *r*, but is rolled	rodilla
RR	doble erre	Trilled *rr* sound. No longer considered a letter by the RAE	socorro HELP!
S	ese	Sounds like an English *s*	sarampión
T	te	Sounds like an English *t but softer*	tos
U	u	Sounds like *oo* in *food* (note that when u is part of dipthong such as ua or ue, it sounds like an English *W*)	urólogo
V	ve or uve; also called ve corta, ve chica, ve de vaca	Sounds like the Spanish *b* (The lips don't touch and there is less aspiration)	vacuna
W	doble ve or uve doble	The letter *W* is not native to the Spanish language, but sounds like the English *w* & only appears in loanwords such as web & watt	síndrome de Down's
X	equis	Sounds like *ks* in English 'socks'	rayo X
Y	ye; also called I griega	Sounds like the *y* in English *yes*. At the end of a words, it sounds like the letter *I* (hay)	yodo
Z	zeta	Sounds like the Englsih *s*; in many parts of Spain it is a *th* sound	zumbido

La Real Academia Española (RAE) or Royal Spanish Academy states that the Spanish alphabet has 27 letters. The Spanish language coincides with the English alphabet except that the Spanish alphabet has one additional letter, ñ (In 2010 RAE eliminated CH and LL as letters in Spanish alphabet).

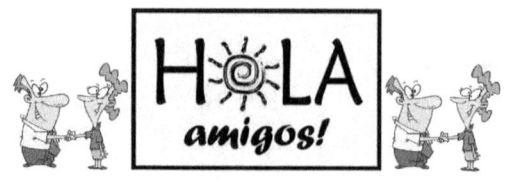

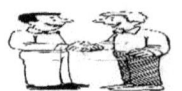

Greetings & Good-byes   Saludos y despedidas

Hello	Hola
Good morning	Buenos días
Good afternoon	Buenas tardes
Good evening	Buenas noches
Until...	Hasta + specific future time frame
	Example: Until next week. Hasta la semana próxima.
See you later	Hasta luego
See you tomorrow	Hasta mañana
See you soon	Hasta pronto or Hasta la vista
Have a nice day	Que tenga un buen día
Goodbye	Adiós/ Chau

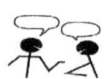

Basic Daily Expressions   Expresiones diarias

What's happening?	¿ Qué tal? ¿Qué pasa?
What's new? What's up?	¿Qué hay de nuevo?
How's it going ? (formal)	¿Cómo le va ?
How's it going ? (familiar)	¿Cómo te va ?

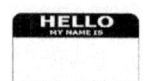

Name   Nombre

What is your name/ last name? (formal)	¿Cómo se llama?
	¿Cuál es su nombre/apellido?
What is your name/ last name? (familiar)	¿Cómo te llamas? ¿Cuál es tu nombre/apellido?

Introductions   Presentaciones
Introducing yourself

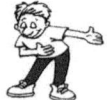

My name is …	Me llamo _____
	Yo soy _____
	Mi nombre es _____

38

Introducing Others

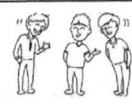

I would like to introduce you to....	Le presento a...(formal)
	Te presento a.. (familiar)
Nice to meet you.	Mucho gusto.
It's a pleasure to meet you. (formal)	Es un placer conocerle.
It's a pleasure to meet you. (familiar)	Es un placer conocerte.
My pleasure.	El placer es mío.
Charmed .	Encantado/a

Nationality / Nacionalidad

Where are you from ? (formal)	¿De dónde es Usted?
Where are you from ? (familiar)	¿De dónde eres tú?
I am from_____.	Yo soy de_____.(country)
	Yo soy_____(nationality)

OJO *take note* : Rules of Thumb for expressing nationality:

Countries are capitalized. Nationalities are not capitalized.
Example: I am from Mexico. Yo soy de México. I am Mexican. Yo soy mexicano/a.
Adjectives of nationality must agree in gender and number with the noun they are refer-ring to. They come after the noun. Example: la comida española (the Spanish food), el restaurante italiano (the Italian restaurant).
The typical endings for adjectives of nationality in Spanish are: *-ano, -ense, -l, -és, -eño,* and *-o.* If the nationality ending is a consonant, add an –a for the feminine version.

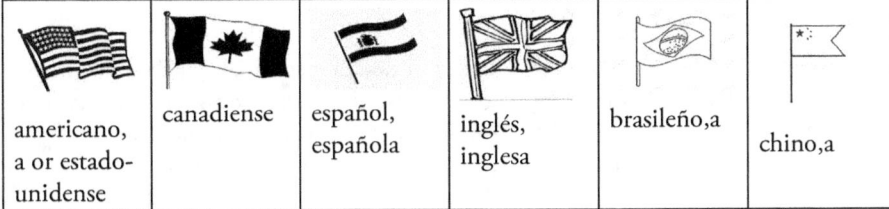

americano, a or estado-unidense	canadiense	español, española	inglés, inglesa	brasileño,a	chino,a

Address / Dirección

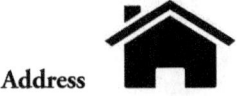

Where do you live? (formal)	¿Dónde vive Usted?
Where do you live? (familiar)	¿Dónde vives?
I live in_____	Yo vivo en _____

Profession/Job

Profesión / trabajo

What do you do? (formal)	¿En qué trabaja? ¿En qué se dedica?
What do you do ? (familiar)	¿En qué trabajas? ¿En qué te dedicas?
I am a _____	Yo soy _____

OJO *take note* : To express someone's line of work use: *SER + occupation or job*. The article is omitted, unless you are adding an adjective to describe the person.

Example: I am a doctor. Yo soy médico, a. I am a kind doctor. Yo soy un médico amable.

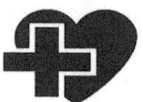

Health

Salud

How are you? (formal)	¿Cómo está Usted?
How are you? (familiar)	¿Cómo estás tú?
I am well .. sick ..regular ..so so	Estoy bien..enfermo(a) ....regular..así así

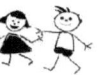

\Looks & Personality Traits

Razcos físicos y razcos de la personalidad

What are you like? (formal)	¿Cómo es Usted?
What are you like? (familiar)	¿Cómo eres tú?
I am _____	Yo soy _____

OJO *take note* : Use the verb **ser** to describe essential qualities or intrinsic characteristics of a person or a thing, such as physical appearance and personality traits.
Example: Juan is tall, handsome and nice. Juan es alto, guapo y simpático.
Ana is blond, pretty and hard-working. Ana es rubia, bonita y trabajadora.

Age

Edad

How old are you ?	¿Cúantos años tiene Usted ? (formal)
	¿Cúantos años tienes tú ? (familiar)
I am _____old.	Yo tengo ___años

OJO *take note* : Age is expressed with the verb **tener** in Spanish. It is one of the many idiomatic expressions with tener. Example: I am 20 years old. Yo tengo veinte años.

Expressions of Courtesy   *Expresiones de cortesía*

Thank you   Gracias
Please   Por favor
You're welcome.   De nada
I'm sorry.   Lo siento.
Pardon me.   Perdón
Excuse me.   Disculpe. Con permiso.
Take care.   Cuídese (formal) Cuídate (familiar).
Bless you!   (after someone sneezes)¡Salud!
Welcome!   ¡Bienvenido(a)!

Days of the week  **Los días de la semana**

Days of the week in Spanish are lower case, masculine and are not pluralized except for Saturday & Sunday. The first day of the week is Monday.

Monday-lunes	Tuesday-martes	Wednesday-miércoles	Thursday-jueves	Friday-viernes	Saturday-sábado	Sunday-domingo

OJO *take note* To express that an action that is being done on a certain day of the week use 'el' example. Yo trabajo el lunes. I work this Monday. To express an action that is repeated use 'los'. Example: Yo trabajo los lunes. I work every Monday.

NUMBERS IN SPANISH:

Cero	Uno	Dos	Tres	Cuatro	Cinco	Seis
0	1	2	3	4	5	6
Siete	Ocho	Nueve	Diez	Once	Doce	Trece
7	8	9	10	11	12	13
Catorce	Quince	Diez y seis or Dieciseis	Diez y siete or diecisiete	Diez y ocho or dieciocho	Diez y nueve or diecinueve	Veinte
14	15	16	17	18	19	20

OJO *take note*: Add the word 'y' to form any numbers past 30. Example: 35 students Treinta y cinco estudiantes.

Thirty- treinta **30**	Forty- cuarenta **40**	Fifty – cincuenta **50**	Sixty- sesenta **60**	Seventy- setenta **70**	Eighty- ochenta **80**	Ninety – noventa **90**	One hundred - cien, ciento **100**

OJO *take note* Numbers in Spanish precede the noun as in English.

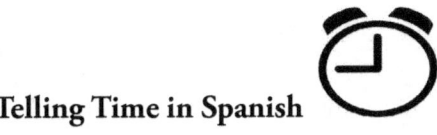

Telling Time in Spanish

What time is it?   **¿Qué hora es?**

¿Qué hora es? Literally means What hour is it? When telling time in Spanish, the word hour (hora) is implied.

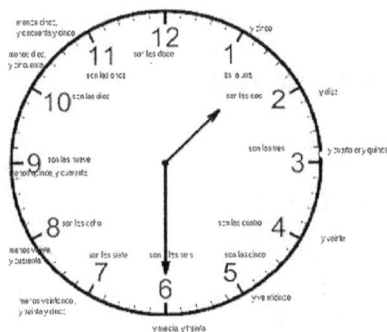

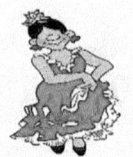

To tell time:

Es la ____ Use for 1:oo o'clock. Example: It is 1:00. Es la una.

Son las _____ Use for any hour greater than 1:00. Example: It is 8:00. Son las ocho.

OJO *take note* **:** The feminine article (*la/las*) is used before the number because it refers to *la hora*.

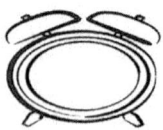 **KEY TIME WORDS:**

Use 'y' (and) to add minutes.
Use 'menos' (less) to subtract minutes.
Use 'en punto' to express 'on the dot'.
Use 'cuarto' or 'quince' to express 15 minutes.
Use 'media' to express half an hour.
Use 'de la mañana' to express AM.
Use 'de la tarde' to express afternoon.
Use 'de la noche' to express PM.
To express time of day use:
- *mediodía* – midday
- *mañana* – in the morning
- *noche* – at night
- *madrugada* – the middle of the night
- *medianoche* – midnight
- *amanecer* – dawn
- *tarde* – in the afternoon

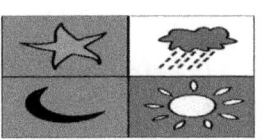

Seasons & Months **Estaciones y meses**

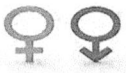 Fall → otoño September → el septiembre October → el octubre November → el noviembre	Winter → invierno December → el diciembre January → el enero February → el febrero	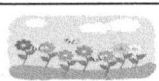 Spring → primavera March → el marzo April → el abril May → el mayo	Summer → verano June → el junio July → el julio August-el agosto

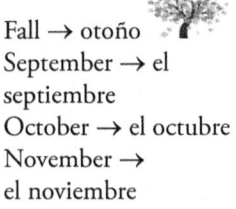 **GENDER & NOUNS IN SPANISH**

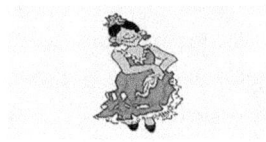

Every noun in Spanish is either masculine or feminine.
BASIC GENDER RULES

| Masculine nouns end in:-O, -N, -R, -S -Y,-PA, -MA, -TA,-AJE
Examples:

--O el libro   el zapato

---N el camión
---AJE el viaje

--R el amor

---S el país

---Y el rey- | Feminine nouns end in: -A, -D (-TAD, -TUD -DAD, -ED), -CION,-SION, -UMBRE
Examples:
---A la mariposa, la cama

--TAD la libertad 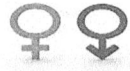

-TUD gratitud

---DAD La ciudad   , -

---ED sed   , |

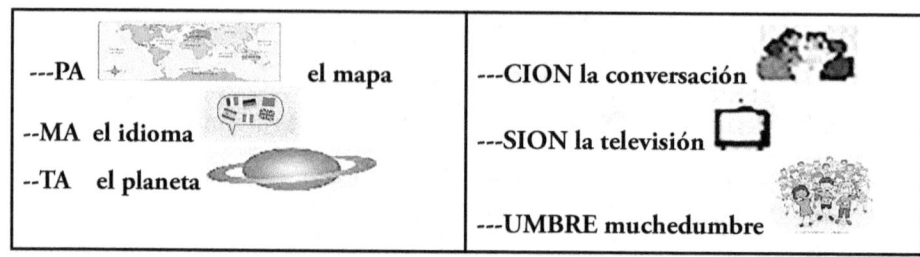

---PA el mapa --MA el idioma --TA el planeta	---CION la conversación ---SION la televisión ---UMBRE muchedumbre

Additional Gender Rules:

♀♀ People or living creatures are referred to by the gender they represent.
Example:el chico la chica

♀♀ Mixed gender- If you are referring to a group of people with mixed gender, you must always use the masculine, even if the ratio of males is less than the ratio of females. Example: los niños

♀♀ Nouns ending in -e and referring to a person can be either masculine or feminine. The article changes depending on the gender of the person, but the noun stays the same. Example: el estudiante la estudiante

♀♀ Nouns that end in *-ista* can be both masculine or feminine. Only the article changes depending on to the gender.
Example:

el turista –the male turist   *la turista – the female tourist*
el dentist-the male dentist   *la dentist*-the female dentist

♀♀ If a masculine noun ends in a consonant, it would have a corresponding female form ending in an *a*.
Example: el profesor → the male professor *a profesora* → the female professor

♀♀ An article can change the meaning of a word. Example: el cura-the priest   la cura-the cure

♀♀ Letters of the alphabet are feminine. Days of the week are masculine.

♀ ♀ **GENDER TRAP:**. Nouns that do not refer to living creatures follow basic gender rules, regardless of whether they are typically associated with males or females. Example: el vestido ▮ la corbata 👔

Feminine Articles

DEFINITE: la, las
INDEFINITE: una, unas

Masculine Articles
DEFINITE: el, los
INDEFINITE: un, unos

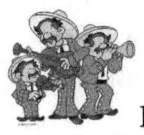

PLURALS IN SPANISH

IF A NOUN ENDS IN A VOWEL: **ADD –S**	IF A NOUN ENDS IN A CONSONANT: **ADD –ES**
IF A NOUN ENDS IN A –Z: **CHANGE TO -CES**	OJO *take note* if a noun is plural, the adjective following it and the article preceding it must also be plurals

POSSESSIVES IN SPANISH

**Possessive adjectives in Spanish go before a noun, as in English.
In Spanish, possessives agree in number with the noun.
The nosotros and vosotros forms also agree in gender.**

PRONOUN	singular	plural	examples
my	mi	mis	mi sombrero🎩my hats, mis sombreros 🎩🎩
your (familiar)	Tu	tus	tu casa🏠 tus casas 🏠🏠
his, hers, your (formal), its	su	sus	su bicicleta🚲 sus bicicletas🚲🚲🚲
our	nuestro, nuestra	nuestros, nuestras	nuestra manzana🍎 nuestras manzanas🍎🍎 nuestro helado 🍦, nuestros helados🍦🍦
your (all) Spain	Vuestro, vuestra	Vuestros, vuestras	vuestra cuchara☐ vuestras cucharas☐☐
Their , your (all) Latin America	su	sus	su hamburguesa🍔, sus hamburguesas🍔🍔

OJO *take note* 'Su' and 'sus' can mean his, hers, yours (formal) its, their or your (plural-Latin America). 'Su' should always be used when the noun is singular and 'sus' should always be used when the noun is plural. example: su casa or sus casas.

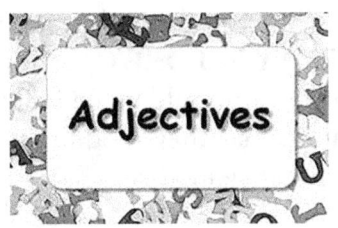

Adjectives

OJO *take note* : Adjectives agree in gender and number with the noun they modify.

angry	Happy	Bored	Nice
![angry face ENOJADO (A)]	![smiley face]	![bored person]	![two nice people]
Enojado/a/os/as	Feliz/felices or Contento/a/os/as	Aburrido/a/os/as	Simpático/a/os/as
Mean/nasty	Smart	Beatiful-lindo/a/os/as	Handsome
![mean figure]	![smart figure]	![beautiful hair]	![handsome man]
Antipático/a/os/as	Inteligente/s	Pretty-bonito/a/os/as	Guapo/a/o/os
Ugly	Fat	Skinny	Tall
![ugly face]	![fat person]	![skinny person]	![tall people]
Feo/a/os/as	Gordo/a/os/as	Delgado/a/os/as	Alto/a/os/as

OJO *take note* : The rule of thumb regarding placement of nouns and adjectives is **QUANTITY BEFORE QUALITY.**

Example: Ten intelligent nurses would be Diez enfermeras/os inteligentes. Adjectives follow the noun that they modify and agree in gender & in number with the noun that they modify.

Demonstrative Adjectives-denote distance of an object or person in relation to the speaker 🌈🌻🌸

Distance from speaker	Masculine singular	Masculine plural	Feminine singular	Feminine plural
Close-this & these	**este**	**estos**	**esta**	**estas**
farther -that & those	**ese**	**esos**	**esa**	**esas**
Farthest-that & those	**aquel**	**aquellos**	**aquella**	**aquellas**

OJO *take note* : If the noun **is not identified**, is **abstract, or is unknown**, the *neuter demonstrative pronouns* **esto, eso**, and **aquello** are used.

Examples: Este libro. This book (CLOSEST TO THE SPEAKER)

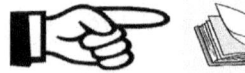

Ese libro. That book. (FURTHER FROM THE SPEAKER)

Aquel libro. That book over there. (FURTHEST FROM THE SPEAKER)

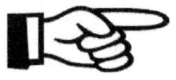 

OJO *take note* : **EASY WAY TO REMEMBER : this & these have the 't's**

QUESTION  **WORDS**

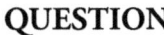

WHO QUIEN (singular) QUIENES (plural)	WHERE DONDE-location	HOW COMO	WHAT/WHICH QUE
HOW MUCH/ HOW MANY CUANTO,A CUANTOS,AS	WHY PORQUE	WHEN CUANDO	WHICH CUAL

OJO *take note* : Some question words can be preceeded by a preposition. This modifies their meaning. Example:

The question word 'quien':

A quien (singular), a quienes (plural): to whom

Con quien (singular), con quienes (plural): with whom

Para quien (singular), para quienes (plural): for whom

De quien (singular), de quienes (plural): whose (possession)

The question word 'donde':

De donde –from where (nationality)

A donde-destination

SPANISH PRONOUN CHART

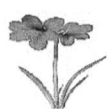

OJO *take note* Pronouns are key to mastering Spanish grammar. Below are 4 **MUST KNOW** types of pronouns in Spanish:

Subject pronouns	Reflexive Pronouns	DOP	IDOP
Yo-I	me	me	me
Tú (you familiar)	te	te	te
Él, ella, Usted	se	lo, la	le
nosotros	nos	nos	nos
vosotros	os	os	os
Ellos, ellas, Uds	se	los,las	les

SUBJECT PRONOUNS

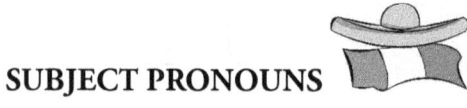

OJO *take note* **In Spanish, subject pronouns are generally used for** emphasis or clarity. Unlike in English, in Spanish you can omit a personal pronoun before a verb. The verb conjugations make clear the subject of the sentence. For example: **Hablas español.** *You speak Spanish.* **Hablamos español.** *We speak Spanish.* The 3rd person singular or plural is where there is room for ambiguity because the 3rd person singular can be he, she, you (formal) or it.

OJO *take note* There is no equivalent translation for the subject pronoun "it" . You simply omit the subject pronoun altogether and use the 3rd person of the verb: **Es bonita.** *It is beautiful.* **Funciona bien.** *It works well.*

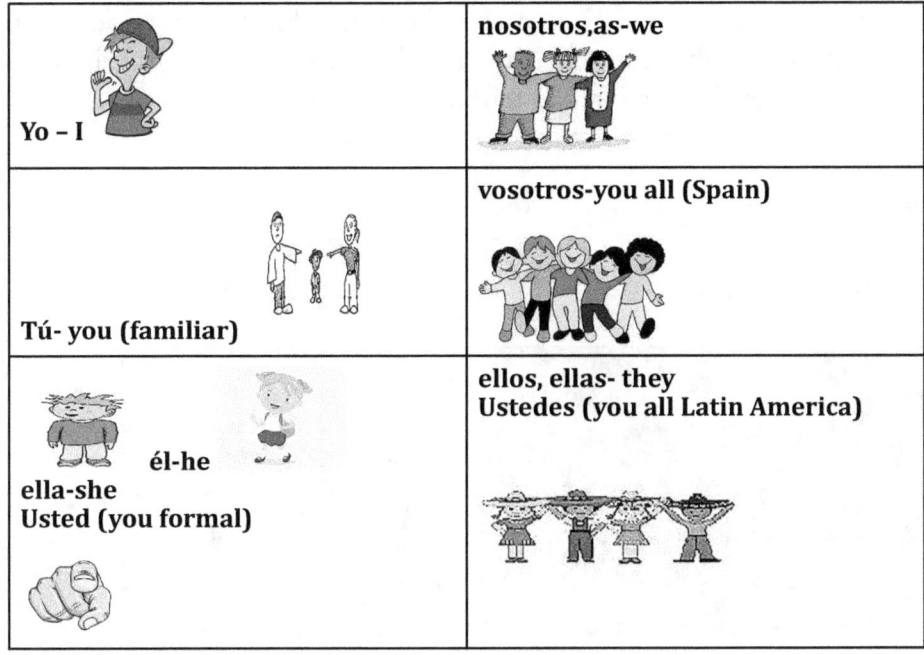

Yo – I	nosotros,as-we
Tú- you (familiar)	vosotros-you all (Spain)
él-he ella-she Usted (you formal)	ellos, ellas- they Ustedes (you all Latin America)

OJO *take note* In Spanish there are two personal pronouns for *"you"* singular: **tú** and **usted.**

Tú is used informally, i.e when talking to a friend, a person we know well, a child, young people and someone that you would address on a first-name basis.

Usted is used formally, i.e when talking to a person you do not know, someone who is older, or someone you are addressing with a title.

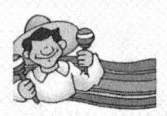

Reflexive Pronouns

OJO *take note* Reflexive verbs reflect back to the person doing the action. They are used only if the subject is doing the action to themselves.

The verb 'lavar' is an example of this concept. It can be used as lavar (non-reflexive) or lavarse (reflexive). The key is who is the subject doing the action to.

Example: I wash the car. Yo lavo el coche. (the subject does the action to the car) Juan washes the pet. Juan lava el mascote. (the subject does the action to the pet) Therefore, no reflexive is needed.

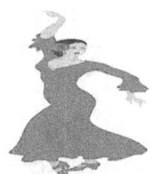

NON REFLEXIVE   **REFLEXIVE**

Yo lavo	Nosotros lavamos	Yo me lavo	Nosotros nos lavamos
Tú lavas	Vosotros laváis	Tú te lavas	Vosotros os laváis
Él, ella, Ud lava	Ellos, ellas, Uds lavan	Él, ella, Usted Se lava	Ellos, ellas, Uds Se lavan

EXAMPLES: I wash myself. Me lavo. Juan washes himself. Juan se lava. We wash ourselves. Nos lavamos. (The subject does the action to themselves).

OJO *take note* Some common reflexive verbs in Spanish are daily routine verbs such as despertarse (to wake up), bañarse- to take a bath, ducharse-to take a shower, maquillarse-to put on makeup, afeitarse- to shave.

Direct & Indirect Object Pronouns

OJO *take note* To figure out which is the direct object and which is the indirect object of a sentence, your starting point is always the **subject and verb of the sentence**.

DOP (Direct Object Pronoun) –Answers the question 'who or what' with regard to the verb. A DOP can be a person, place or thing. Ex. I read the book. I read it. Julia loves Miguel. Julia loves him

DOP Rules of Thumb:

In English the order is verb +DOP. In Spanish the order is DOP + verb for simple sentences (the rule changes when you have 2 verbs together)

Example: Juan lee el libro. Juan **lo** lee. Juan reads the book. Juan reads it.

IDOP (Indirect Object Pronoun)-Aswers the question '**to whom, for whom**' with regard to the verb and is usually found at the end of the sentence. IDOPs always refer to a person. Example: Jorge buys the book for Juan. Jorge buys the book for him.

IDOP Rules of Thumb:

In English the order is verb + IDOP. In Spanish, the order is IDOP + verb. (the rule changes when you have 2 verbs together)

Example: Juan reads the book to Geraldo. Juan **le** lee el libro.

OJO *take note* The 3ʳᵈ person 'le' can mean to him, to her, to you (formal) or to it (such as a pet). You can use context to figure out who it is referring to or you add a clarifier to a sentence Example-Yo le doy la computadora a Jorge. The clarifier ' a Jorge', lets the reader know that 'le' in this case, is to him or to Jorge.

Direct & Indirect Object Pronouns TOGETHER

In Spanish, as in English, you can use both DOPs & IDOPs in a sentence together .

DOP & IDOP TOGETHER Rules of Thumb:

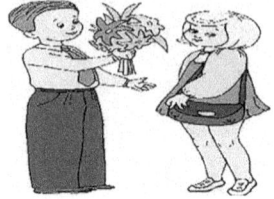

SPANISH: IDOP + DOP + verb (English: verb + DOP + IDOP)

DOP-answers the question 'what or who'

IDOP-answers the question 'to whom'

Juan gives flowers to me. Juan gives them to me.

Juan da las flores a mí. Juan me las da.

OJO *take note* In English, the order for IDOP & DOPs used together is verb+DOP+IDOP . In Spanish the order is IDOP+DOP+verb for simple sentences (the rule changes when you have 2 verbs together).

Example. I read the book to you (familiar). I read it to you. Yo **te lo** leo.

OJO *take note* **In Spanish you can never have an indirect and direct object that both start with an 'l'. You must substitute the indirect object with the pronoun 'se'. Example- Yo doy el libro a Juan. Yo le lo doy is incorrect. You must say: Yo se lo doy.**

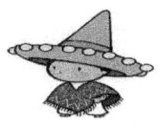

SPANISH: IDOP + DOP + verb (English: verb + DOP + IDOP)

DOP-answers the question 'what or who'

IDOP-answers the question 'to whom'

Juan gives flowers to Marta. Juan gives them to her.

Juan da las flores a Marta. Juan le las da IS INCORRECT. 'LE' becomes 'SE'. CORRECT ANSWER: Juan se las da.

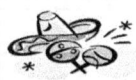 **VERBS –In Spanish there are 3 types of verbs: -ar, -er, -ir**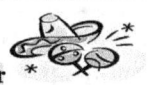

REGULAR VERB ENDINGS FOR –AR, -ER & -IR VERBS

OJO *take note* The subject or subject pronoun determines which ending to use.

Subject Pronoun	Habl-ar	Com-er	Viv-ir
Yo	Habl-o	Com-o	Viv-o
Tú	Habl-as	Com-es	Viv-es
Él, ella, Usted	Habl-a	Com-e	Viv-e
Nosotros	Habl-amos	Com-emos	Viv-imos
Vosotros	Habl-áis	Com-éis	Viv-ís
Ellos, ellas, Ustedes	Habl-an	Com-en	Viv-en

OJO (*take note* Vosotros (you all-addressing a group of people) is used in Spain and Ustedes (you all-plural), is used in Latin America. You may hear a variation of vosotros in Argentina or Colombia, ex -Vos trabajás (you work).

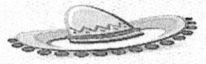

SER VS ESTAR –In Spanish, there are two verbs that mean 'to be' .

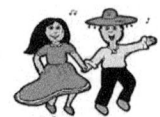

SER   **ESTAR**

Yo soy	Yo estoy
Tú eres	Tú estás
Él, ella, Usted es	Él, ella, Usted está
Nosotros somos	Nosotros estamos
Ellos,ellas, Ustedes son	Ellos,ellas, Ustedes estan

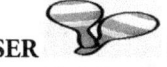

SER **SER-used for situations considered permanent**

DATE
Example: Today is Monday, January 15th. Hoy es lunes, el quince de enero.

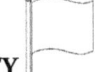

OCCUPATION
Example: I am a teacher. Yo soy profesor,a.

TIME ☺☺☽
Example: It is 9:00am . Son las nueve de la mañana.

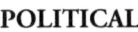

NATIONALITY
Example: The students are American. Los estudiantes son americanos.

AFFILIATION- RELIGIOUS OR

POLITICAL
Example: I am a Democrat. Yo soy demócrata. He is a Republican. El es republicano. Felipe is Catholic. Felipe es católico. Ruben is Jewish. Rubén es judio.

CHARACTERISTIC - intrinsic or essential characteristics that define the essence of someone or something.
Example: Carmen is inteligente. Carmen es inteligente. The bicycle is made of metal. La bicicleta es de metal.

POSSESSION OR OWNERSHIP.
Example: It is Juan's house. La casa es de Juan.

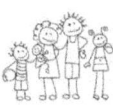

RELATIONSHIP
Example: Miguel is Ana's uncle. Miguel es el tío de Ana.

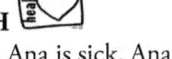 **ESTAR-used for temporary, or changeable situations (acronym-HELP)**

• **HEALTH**
• Example: Ana is sick. Ana está enferma.
• **EMOTIONS OR MOOD** 😩😫, ☺
  Example: Jorge is sad. Jorge está triste.

• **LOCATION**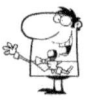
  Example: Maria is in Madrid. Maria está en Madrid.
• **P=Present progressive**
• Example: I am speaking with Jorge.
  Estoy hablando con Jorge.

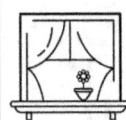

• **P= present temporary condition**
  Example:
  The window is open. La ventana está abierta.

OJO *take note* Ser & estar both have different uses .They can not be interchanged without affecting the meaning.

To be boring- Ser aburrido/a	To be bored -Estar abur- rido/a
To be clever -Ser listo/a	To be ready- Estar listo/a **Ready**
To be conceited -Ser orgulloso/a	To be proud- Estar orgulloso/a
To be rich -Ser rico/a	To be tasty- Estar rico/a
To be safe- Ser seguro/a SAFETY FIRST	To be certain -Estar seguro/a
To be bad- Ser malo	To be ill- Estar malo

PREPOSITIONS OF LOCATION

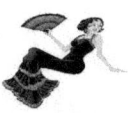

In front of Enfrente de, delante de Los libros están delante del chico.	*Next to Al lado de* El perro está al lado del hombre.	To the left *A la izquierda de* La niña está sentada a la izquierda del pupitre.	To the right *A la derecha de* La niña está sentada a la derecha del pupitre.
Under *debajo de* *La pelota está debajo de la mesa*	*Around* *Alrededor de* La familia está alrededor de la mesa.	*On/upon Sobre* Los libros están sobre la mesa.	Between *Entre* El plato está entre la cuchara y el tenedor.
Inside dentro de El niño está dento de la caja.	Behind *Detrás de* La pizarra está detrás del profesor.	Close to - *Cerca de* . El hombre está cerca de la mujer.	Far from *Lejos de* El chico está lejos de la casa.

OJO *take note* **Prepositions of location are used with the verb estar**

IR – to go	OJO *take note* IR + A + INFINITIVE is a future construction used to express a future action. Ex- Voy a trabajar. I am going to work
Yo voy	Nosotros vamos
Tú vas	Vosotros vaís
Él, ella, Ud va	Ellos, ellas, Ustedes van
TENER-to have	OJO: *take note* Tener has many idiomatic expressions such as : Tener frío-to be cold, tener calor-to be hot, tener __ años-to be __ years old Tener + que+ INFINITIVE= To have to do something
Yo tengo	Nosotros tenemos
Tú tienes	Vosotros tenéis
Él, ella, Usted tiene	Ellos, ellas, Ustedes tienen

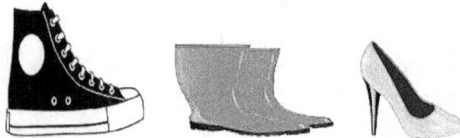

STEM CHANGING VERBS -also referred to as
SHOE, BOOT, SNEAKER VERBS.

There are 4 different types: **o:ue, e:ie, e:i, u:ue (jugar-to play-is the only u:ue stem-changing verb).**

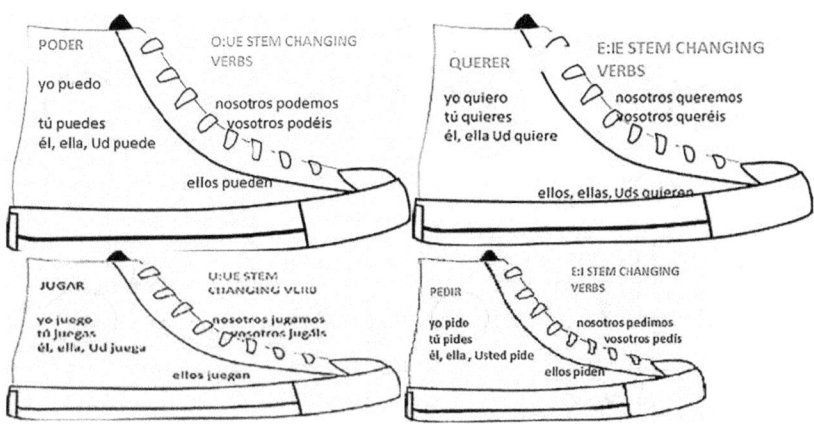

OJO *take note* The stem-changing verbs are classified as shoe/boot/sneaker verbs to facilitate learning their conjugations for the beginner student. Shoe verbs have stem changes in every form except nosotros & vosotros. They are classified as shoe verbs because both nosotros & vosotros are outside of the shoe. All regular forms are outside the shoe.

👣👣 GO VERBS -Verbs that have a go ending in the yo form
The Spanish "yo-go" verbs are as follows:

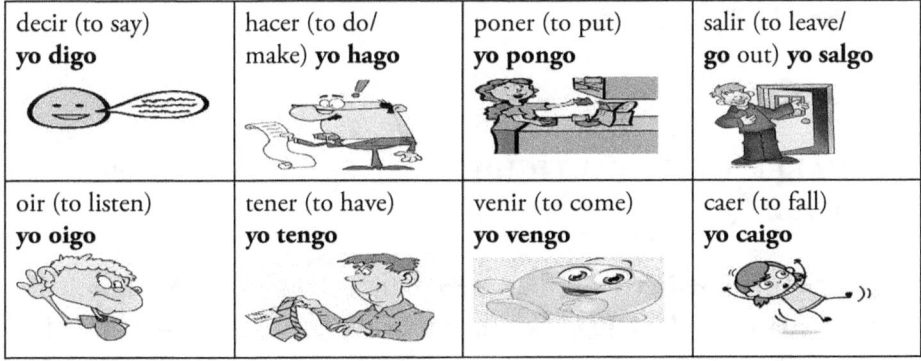

decir (to say) **yo digo**	hacer (to do/ make) **yo hago**	poner (to put) **yo pongo**	salir (to leave/ go out) **yo salgo**
oir (to listen) **yo oigo**	tener (to have) **yo tengo**	venir (to come) **yo vengo**	caer (to fall) **yo caigo**

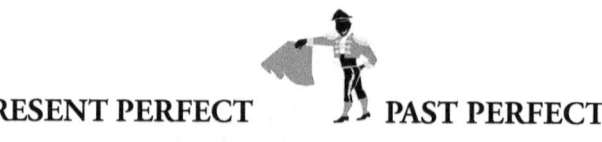

PRESENT PERFECT   PAST PERFECT

HABER-auxiliary verb

Yo	he	había
Tú	has	habías
Él, ella, Usted	ha	había
Nosotros	hemos	habíamos
Vosotros	habéis	habíais
Ellos, Ellas, Ustedes	han	habían

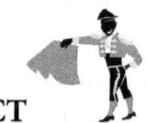

PRESENT PERFECT

USE HABER + PAST PARTICIPLE (-ado for –ar verbs & -ido for -ir & -er verbs) Example: Juan ha comido. Juan has eaten. Yo he llamado a Juan. I have called Juan. Tú has vivido en México. You have lived in Mexico

PAST PERFECT

USE HABER + PAST PARTICIPLE (-ado for –ar verbs & -ido for -ir & -er verbs)

Example: Juan había comido. Juan had eaten. Yo había llamado a Juan. I called Juan. Tú habías vivido en México. You had lived in Mexico

PAST TENSE- PRETERIT & IMPERFECT

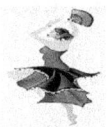

PRETERIT

Subject Pronoun	Habl-ar	Com-er	Viv-ir
Yo	Habl-é	Com-í	Viv-í
Tú	Habl-aste	Com-iste	Viv-iste
Él, ella, Usted	Habl-ó	Com-ió	Viv-ió
Nosotros	Habl-amos	Com-imos	Viv-imos
Vosotros	Habl-asteis	Com-isteis	Viv-isteis
Ellos, ellas, Ustedes	Habl-aron	Com-ieron	Viv-ieron

OJO *take note* The preterit tense has two sets of endings: one for –ar verbs and the same for –er & -ir verbs for regular verbs. The nosotros for –ar is the same in the present tense and the preterit tense. Context determines which tense it is referring to. Ex-Hablamos con Juan todos los días- We speak with Juan every day. Ayer hablamos con Juan. We spoke with Juan yesterday.

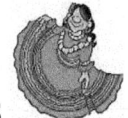

PRETERIT IRREGULARS

	yo	tú	Él, ella, Usted	Nosotros, nosotras	Ellos, ellas, Ustedes
IR & SER	fui	Fuiste	fue	fuimos	fueron
DAR	di	diste	dio	dimos	dieron
VER	vi	viste	Vio	vimos	vieron

OJO *take note* Ir and ser have the same preterit conjugation. Context determines which is being used. Ex-Juan fue al cine. Juan went to the movies. Juan fue simpático. Juan was nice.

U-STEM PRETERIT IRREGULARS✿

ESTAR (u-stem)	estuve	estuviste	estuvo	estuvimos	estuvieron
TENER (u-stem)	tuve	tuviste	tuvo	tuvimos	tuvieron
ANDAR (u-stem)	anduve	anduviste	anduvo	anduvimos	anduvieron
PONER- (u-stem)	puse	pusiste	puso	pusimos	pusieron
SABER (u-stem)	supe	supiste	supo	supimos	supieron
PODER (u-stem)	pude	pudiste	pudo	pudimos	pudieron

I-STEM PRETERIT IRREGULARS✿

HACER (I-stem)	Hice	hiciste	hizo	hicimos	hicieron
QUERER (I-stem)	quise	quisiste	quiso	quisimos	quisieron
VENIR (I-stem)	vine	viniste	vino	vinimos	vinieron

J-STEM PRETERIT IRREGULARS✿

DECIR	dije	dijiste	dijo	dijimos	dijeron
TRAER	traje	trajiste	trajo	trajimos	trajeron
CONDUCIR	conduje	condujiste	condujo	condujimos	condujeron

OJO *take note* The preterit has various irregular verbs. Among them are the : u-stem, i-stem and j-stem. The verbs endings for the i, j and u stem verbs are: -e. -iste, -o, -imos, -isteis and-ieron. There are no accents on any of the preterit -i,-j or –u stems. The –j stems 3rd person plural form is –eron. The 3rd person singular for hacer is hizo.

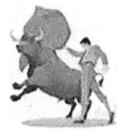

IMPERFECT

Subject Pronoun	Habl-ar	Com-er	Viv-ir
Yo	Habl-aba	Com-ía	Viv-ía
Tú	Habl-abas	Com-ías	Viv-ías
Él, ella, Usted	Habl-aba	Com-ía	Viv-ía
Nosotros	Habl-ábamos	Com-íamos	Viv-íamos
Vosotros	Habl-abais	Com-iais	Viv-iais
Ellos, ellas, Ustedes	Habl-aban	Com-ían	Viv-ían

OJO *take note* The first & third person conjugations are the same in the imperfect. If the subject or subject pronoun is not listed, context will help you determine subject.

IRREGULAR IMPERFECT

Subject Pronoun	Ir	Ser	ver
Yo	iba	era	Veía
Tú	ibas	eras	Veías
Él, ella, Usted	iba	era	Veía
Nosotros	íbamos	eramos	Veíamos
Vosotros	ibáis	erais	Veiais
Ellos, ellas, Ustedes	iban	eran	Veían

OJO *take note* The imperfect has only 3 irregulars: ir, ser and ver.

PRETERIT VS IMPERFECT USES ❦

PRETERIT❁ past completed action with a clear beginning & a clear end. Ex Yesterday I studied. Ayer estudié.	IMPERFECT❁ past repeated action, background action, time, age, whenever you would say 'was' or 'used to' in English Ex Cuando era niño, estudiaba todos los días. When I was a kid, I used to study every day.
ACRONYM FOR CHOOSING BETWEEN PRETERIT VS IMPERFECT **SIMBA CHEATED** PRETERIT- **SIMBA** (**S**ingle Action, **I**nterruption, **M**ain Event, **B**eginning Action, **A**rrivals/Departures) IMPERFECT- **CHEATED** (**C**haracteristics, **H**ealth, **E**motion, **A**ge, **T**ime, **E**ndless activities, **D**ate)	

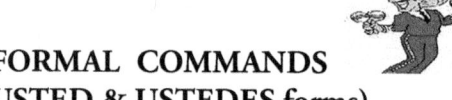

FORMAL COMMANDS   (**Formal command have only**
USTED & USTEDES forms)

OJO *take note* **Go to the 'yo' form of a verb, drop the –o and add the opposite vowel (-e for –ar verbs & -a for –er and –ir verbs)**

SUBJECT	comprar	vender	escribir
USTED	compr-e	venda	escriba
USTEDES	compr-en	vendan	escriban

There are 6 irregular Ud/Uds commands: dar - to give: dé, den.

- estar - to be. esté, estén
- haber - to have (auxiliary verb) haya, hayan
- ir - to go. vaya, vayan
- saber - to know. sepa, sepa.
- ser - to be. sea, sean

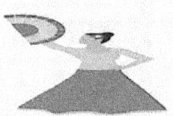

THE PRESENT SUBJUNCTIVE

OJO To form the present subjunctive: go to the 'yo' form of a verb, drop the –o and add the opposite vowel (-e for –ar verbs & -a for –er and –ir verbs).

Subject Pronoun	Habl-ar	Com-er	Viv-ir
Yo	Habl-e	Com-a	Viv-a
Tú	Habl-es	Com-as	Viv-as
Él, ella, Usted	Habl-e	Com-a	Viv-a
Nosotros	Habl-emos	Com-amos	Viv-amos
Vosotros	Habl-eis	Com-ais	Viv-ais
Ellos, ellas, Ustedes	Habl-en	Com-an	Viv-an

OJO The present subjunctive is used when there are 2 separate clauses in a sentence and used when there is **wish, emotion or doubt ACRONYM: WEDDING**.

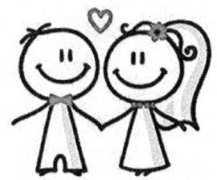

example-

WISH: I want Juan to study . Quiero que Juan estudie.

EMOTION: I hope Juan studies. Espero que Juan estudie.

DOUBT: I doubt that Juan will study. Dudo que Juan estudie.

GLOSSARY OF DENTAL TERMS

Abcess	absceso
AIDS	SIDA
Allergic	alérgico/a
Allergy	alérgia
Alleviate	aliviar
Amalgam	amalgama
Anesthetic	anestético
Antibiotics	antibiótico
Appointment	cita
Artificial	artificial/ postizo
Baby tooth	diente de leche
Bear pain	aguantar
Biopsy	biopsia
Bite	morder
Bleach	blanquear
Bleed	sangrar
Blood	sangre
Bone	hueso
Bother	molestar
Breath	aliento
Breathe	respirar
Bridge	puenet

Broken	quebrado, roto
Brush	cepillo, cepillarse (verb)
Canine	lomillo
Cavity	caries
Chronic	crónico
Composite	resina
Crown	corona
Decayed	picado, deteriorado
Dentis	dentista
Denture	dentadura postiza
Enamel	esmalte
Esthetic	estético.a
Filling	relleno, empaste
Floss	seda dental, hilo dental, usar el hilo dental-to use floss
Fluoride	fluoruro
Gum	encía
Health	salud
Hot	caliente
Ice	hielo
Illness	enfermedad
Impression	impresión, molde
Infected	infectado
Injection	inyección
Injured	lastimado, a

Jaw	mandíbula
Lip	labio
Lukewarm	tibio
Mask	cubreboca
Medicine	medicina
Mirror	espejo
Molar	molar
Mouth	boca
Needle	aguja
Nerve	nervio
Pregnant	embarazada
Pressure	presión
Radiograph	radiografía, placa de rayos X
Refer	referir
Remove	quitar
Restoration	restauración
Rinse	enjuague
root	raíz
Saliva	saliva
Salivary gland	glándula salivar
Scale	raspar
Sensitive	sensitivo,a
Silver	plata
Smile	sonrisa, sonreír (verb)

Stitch	puntada
Straighten	enderezar
Surgery	cirugía
Suture	sutura, suturar (v)
Swell	inflamar, hichar
Symptom	síntoma
Syringe	jeringa
Tissue	tejido
Tongue	lengua
Tonsils	amígdalas
Tooth	diente
Toothpaste	pasta dental
Ulcer	úlcera
Wisdom teeth	muelas del juicio
wound	herida
X-rays	rayos X

PRACTICE EXERCISES

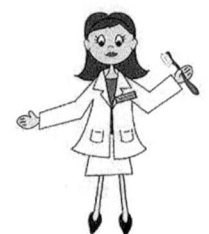

RECEPTIONIST/ RECEPTIONISTA

1. Ask a patient for his/her first and last name.

_____

2. Ask a patient for his/her date of birth.

_____

3. Ask a patient for his/her marital status.

_____

4. Ask a patient to fill out a form.

_____

5. Ask a patient to take a seat and to wait for a moment.

_____

6. Tell a patient that you will attend to him shortly.

_____

DENTAL TEAM. Please choose the correct answer.

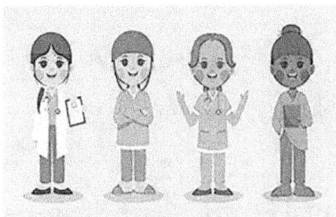

1. Dental Assistant
2. Dental Technician
3. Dentist
4. Endodontist /root canal specialist
5. Hygienist
6. Implant Specialist
7. Oral surgeon
8. Orthodontist/Brace specialist
9. Periodontist / gum specialist
10. Prosthodontist/denture specialist
11. Receptionist

A. el/la recepcionista
B. Prostodontista/especialista en dentaduras
C. especialista de implantes
D. ortodoncista/especialista de frenillos
E. especialista en encías / periodontista
F. el dentista / la dentista
G. el/la técnico (a) dental
H. endodontista / especialista en canal radicular
I. el/la higienista
J. el cirujano oral
K. el/la asistente

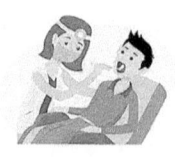

Los dientes Match the pictures to the Spanish vocabulary.

A. 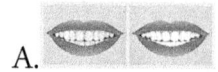 bleaching B. 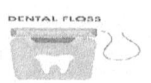 dental floss C. 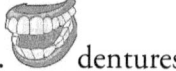 dentures

D. 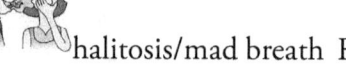 braces E.  halitosis/mad breath F. 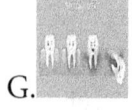 crooked teeth

G. 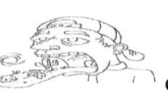 periodontitis H. 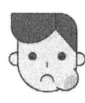 dry mouth I. 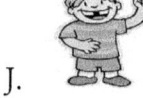 swelling

J. 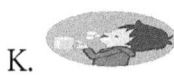 loose tooth

K. 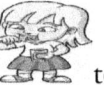 to gargle L. 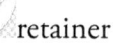 to brush your teeth M. retainer

N. 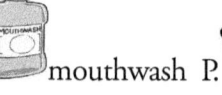 baby tooth O. 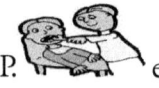 mouthwash P. extract a tooth

Q. 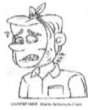 sensitive teeth R. 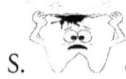 tooth ache

S.  cavity T. 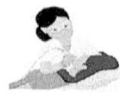 chipped tooth U. root canal /endodontics

_____ 1. enjuague bucal

_____ 2. dientes sensibles

_____ 3. sacarle una muela

_____ 4. diente quebrado

_____ 5. blanqueamiento

_____ 6. hacer gárgaras

_____ 7. periodontitis

_____ 8. halitosis/ el mal aliento crónico

_____ 9. dentadura

_____ 10. endodoncia

_____ 11. cepillarse los dientes

_____ 12. diente flojo

_____ 13. carie

_____ 14. hilo dental

_____ 15. hinchazón

_____ 16. frenos

_____ 17. retenedor

_____ 18. dolor de la muela

_____ 19. diente de la leche

_____ 20. boca seca

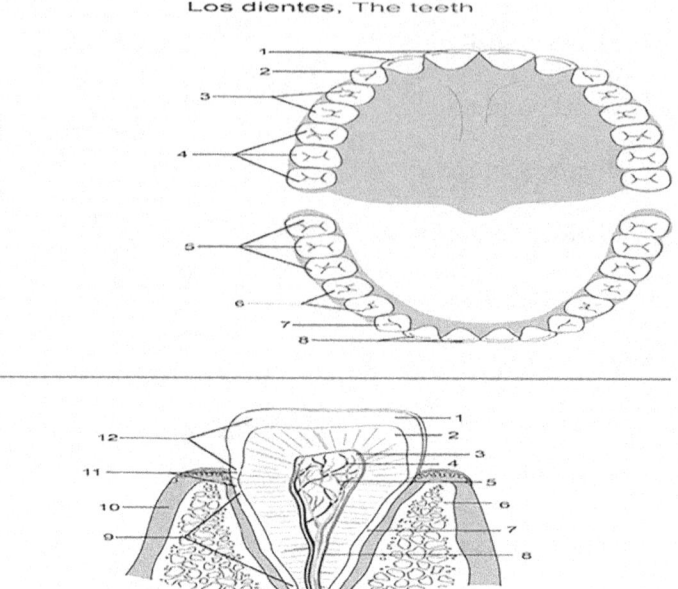

Los dientes, The teeth

La cabeza. Please label each part of the head using the word bank.

el paladar, el pelo/el cabello, los labios, las amígdalas, la pupila, la garganta, el cuero cabelludo, la lengua, el diente, los pómulos, la lengua, el tabique, el párpado, la pestaña, el seno, la córnea, el mentón/la barbilla, las narices, la fosa nasal, la ceja, el iris

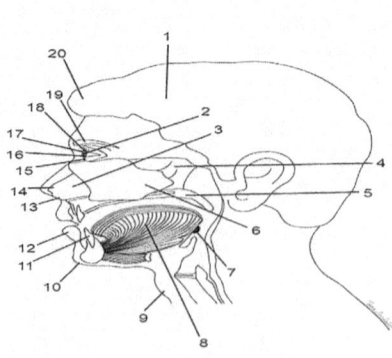

La cabeza, The head

THE MOUTH-LA BOCA Please label each part of the mouth using the word bank.

> La lengua, el labio superior, el arco palatofaríngeo, el paladar duro, la úvula, la encía, la amígdala,palatina, el freno labial superior, el rafe palatino, el arco otofaringe, el palatoglossal, el frenillo lingual, el labio inferior, el paladar blando,el frenillo labia inferior, el vestíbulo, los conductos de la glándula submandibular

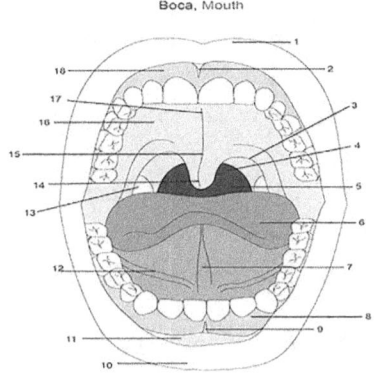

Boca, Mouth

GRAMMAR EXERCISES

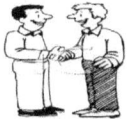

Greetings. Match the Spanish with the correct English translation.

_____Buenos días	A. And you (formal)?
_____Buenas tardes	B. I am from..
_____Buenas noches	C. Thank you
_____¿Qué tal?	D. What is your last name?
_____Hasta mañana	E. Where are you from?
_____Hasta luego	F. Good morning
_____¿Cómo se llama?	G. How are things?
_____¿Cómo está Usted?	H. My name is…
_____¿ De dónde es Usted?	I. Good afternoon
_____¿Cómo se siente?	J. What is your name?

79

_____Yo soy de..   K. And you (familiar)?

_____¿Cuál es su apellido?   L. How are you?

_____Yo estoy bien   M. Good night

_____Me llamo…   N. You're welcome

_____¿ Y tú?   O. Hello

_____¿ Y Usted?   P. See you tomorrow (until tomorrow)

_____Gracias   Q. See you later.

_____De nada   R. How do you feel?

_____Hola   S. I am well

Question Words. Please choose the correct answer.(1 point each = 10 pts)

1 ¿Por qué? Means..a) Who b)What c)Why d)How

2 ¿Cómo? Means...a)How b)What c)Where d)Why e)Who

3. ¿Dónde? means...a)Who b)What c)How d)Where

4. ¿Cuándo? Means...a)When b)Why c)Who d)Where

5. ¿Quién/Quiénes? Means...a)Why b)How c)When d)Who

6. ¿Qué? means...a)Who b) What c)When d)Where

7. ¿Cuánto? means...a)Why b)When c)At what time d)How much/many

8. ¿Cuál/Cuáles? means...a)How? b)Where? c)Who? d)Which?

9. ¿De dónde? means...a)Where (nationality) b)What c)How d)Where (location)

10. ¿A Dónde? means...a)Where (nationality) b)What c)How d)Where (destination)

PRESENT TENSE VERBS TABLE. Please fill in the missing conjugations.

comer	hablar	vivir	tener	ir	ser	estar
Yo como				Yo voy		Yo estoy
	Tú hablas		Tú tienes		Tú eres	
Él, ella, Ud come		Él vive		Él, ella, Ud va		Él, ella, Ud es
	Nosotros hablamos		Nosotros tenemos		Nosotros somos	
		Vostotros vivís		Vosotros váis		
			Ellos tienen			Ellos están

PRETERIT. Please fill in the correct conjugations

1. ESTAR   a) Juan _____ b) nosotros _____ c) yo _____
2. QUERER a) tú _____ b) Jamie y yo _____ c) vosotros _____
3. TRAER   a) Juan y Jorge _____ b) nosotros _____ c) el paciente _____
4. VENIR a) tú _____ b) vosotros _____ c) ellos_____
5. TENER a) tú _____ b) Jamie y yo _____ c) yo _____
6. SER a) Juan _____ b) nosotros _____ c) yo_____
7. IR a) Los estudiantes _____ b) nosotros _____ c) yo _____
8. PODER a) tú _____ b) yo _____ c) ellos_____
9. HACER a) tú _____ b) nosotros _____ c) ellos_____
10. DAR a) tú _____ b) yo _____ c) ellos_____

IMPERFECT VERB TABLE. Please fill in the missing conjugations.

comer	hablar	vivir	tener	ir	ser	ver
Yo comía				Yo iba		Yo veía
	Tú hablabas		Tú tenías		Tú eras	
Él, ella, Ud comía		Él, ella, Ud vivía		Él, ella, Ud iba		Él, ella, Ud veía

Nosotros hablába- mos		Nosotros teníamos		Nosotros éramos	
	Vostotros vivíais		Vosotros ibáis		
		Ellos, ellas, Uds tenían			Ellos veían

PRETERIT VS IMPERFECT Choose between preterit vs imperfect.

1) Yesterday it was raining a lot (weather)Ayer _____ (llovía, llovió)mucho.

2) Every day I worked in the hospital. Todos los días yo _____(trabajé, trabajaba) en el hospital.

3) Last night there was an accident near the hospital. Anoche _____(hubo, había) un accidente cerca del hospital.

4) Juan's car crashed with a truck. El coche de Juan _____ (chocó, chocaba) con un camión (truck).

5. I immediately called 911. Yo inmediatamente _____ (llamé, llamaba) a 911.

6. Juan was unconscious .Juan _____ (estaba, estuvo) insconciente.

7. _____ The ambulance came immediately and they took him to the hospital. La ambulancia_____ (vino, venía) inmediatamente y lo _____ (llevaron, llevaban) al hospital.

8. _____ When I was young, I used to have a lot of car accidents. De joven, _____ (tuve, tenía) muchos choques.

9. _____ Jorge always used to work at the emergency clinic. Jorge siempre _____ (trabajó, trabajaba) en la clínica de emergencia.

10. _____ Yesterday I went to the dentist. Ayer _____ (fui, iba) al dentista.

Ser vs estar. Please choose ser or estar in the following sentences.

1. El hospital _____ (es, está) en Puerto Rico (location)
2. El enfermero _____(es, está) inteligente y simpático (temperament)
3. El paciente _____(es, está) enfermo (health)
4. El dolor _____(es, está) constant (description)
5. Los médicos _____ (son, están) tristes hoy. (mood)

6. Juan _____(es, está) enfermero (occupation)
7. El estetoscopio _____ (es, está) del Dr. López (possession)
8. La bata (gown) _____ (es, está) es de algodón (cotton) (what something is made of)
9. Yo _____(soy, estoy) en el laboratorio (location)
10. Nosotros _____(somos, estamos) aburridos (mood).

ANSWERS

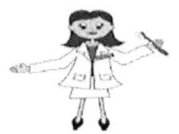

RECEPTIONIST/ RECEPTIONISTA

NOTE: USE THE USTED FORM TO ADDRESS A PATIENT UNLESS OTHERWISE REQUESTED BY THE PATIENT. ANSWERS WILL VARY.

1. Ask a patient for his/her first and last name.
   ¿Cuál es su nombre/apellido (nombre complete)?
2. Ask a patient for his/her date of birth.
   ¿Cuál es su fecha de nacimiento?
3. Ask a patient for his/her marital status.
   ¿Cuál es su estado civil?
4. Ask a patient to fill out a form.
   Llene la planilla, por favor.
5. Ask a patient to take a seat and to wait for a moment.
   Tome asiento por favor y espere un momento.
6. Tell a patient that you will attend to him shortly.
   Le atiendo en seguida OR Enseguida le atiendo.

DENTAL TEAM. Please choose the correct answer.

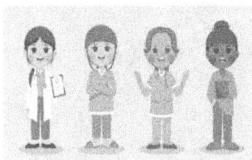

1.	Dental Assistan	K
2.	Dental Technician	G
3.	Dentist	F
4.	Endodontist /root canal specialis	H
5.	Hygienist	I
6.	Implant Specialist	C
7.	Oral surgeon	J
8.	Orthodontist/Brace specialist	D
9.	Periodontist / gum specialist	E
10.	Prosthodontist/denture specialist	B
11.	Receptionist	A

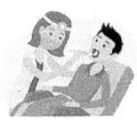

Los dientes Match the pictures to the Spanish vocabulary.

_____ 1. O
_____ 2. Q
_____ 3. P
_____ 4. T
_____ 5. A
_____ 6. K
_____ 7. G
_____ 8. E
_____ 9. C
_____ 10. U
_____ 11. L
_____ 12. J

_____ 13. S
_____ 14. B
_____ 15. I
_____ 16. D
_____ 17. M
_____ 18. R
_____ 19. N
_____ 20. H

Los dientes, The teeth

1. incisivos, incisors
2. canino, canine
3. premolares, premolars
4. molares, molars
5. molares, molars
6. premolares, premolars
7. canino, canine
8. incisivos, incisors

---

1. esmalte, enamel
2. dentina, dentin
3. vena, vein
4. artería, artery
5. nervio, nerve
6. hueso, bone
7. cemento, cementum
8. pulpa, pulp
9. raíz, root
10. encía, gum
11. cuello, neck
12. corona, crown

La cabeza, The head

1. el cuero cabelludo, scalp
2. la pupila/la niña del ojo, pupil
3. la fosa nasal, nasal cavity
4. el seno, sinus
5. el paladar, palate
6. los pómulos, cheekbone
7. las amígdalas/las anginas, tonsils
8. la lengua, tongue
9. la garganta, throat
10. **el mentón/la barbilla**, chin
11. el diente, tooth
12. los labios, lips
13. **las narices/las ventanas de la nariz**, nostrils
14. el tabique, septum
15. el párpado, eyelid
16. el iris, iris
17. la córnea, cornea
18. la pestaña, eyelash
19. la ceja, eyebrow
20. el pelo, el cabello, hair

Boca, Mouth

1. labio superior, upper lip
2. frenillo labial superior, superior labial frenulum
3. palatoglosal, palatoglossal arch
4. palatofaríngeo, palato pharyngealarch
5. orofaringe, oropharynx
6. lengua, tongue
7. frenillo lingual, lingual frenulum
8. encía, gum
9. frenillo labia inferior, labial frenulum
10. labio inferior, lower lip
11. vestíbulo, vestibule
12. conductos de la glándula submandibular, palatine tonsil duct of the sublingual gland
13. amígdala palatina, palatine tonsil
14. úvula, uvula
15. paladar blando, soft palate
16. paladar duro, hard palate
17. afe palatino, alatine raphe
18. encia, gum

GRAMMAR EXERCISES

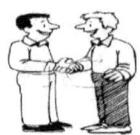

Greetings. Match the Spanish with the correct English translation.

_F_____Buenos días

_I_____Buenas tardes

_M_____Buenas noches

_G_____¿Qué tal?

_P_____Hasta mañana

_Q_____Hasta luego

_J_____¿Cómo se llama?

_R_____¿Cómo está Usted?

_E_____¿ De dónde es Usted?

__R_____¿Cómo se siente?

__B_____Yo soy de..

__D_____¿Cuál es su apellido?

__S_____Yo estoy bien

__H_____Me llamo…

__K_____¿ Y tú?

__A_____¿ Y Usted?

__C_____Gracias

__N_____De nada

__O_____Hola

Question Words. ANSWERS

1¿Por qué?   c)Why

2 ¿Cómo?   a)How

3.¿Dónde?   d)Where

4. ¿Cuándo?   a)When

5. ¿Quién/Quiénes?   d)Who

6.¿Qué?   b) What

7.¿Cuánto?   d)How much/many

8.¿Cuál/Cuáles?   d)Which?

9. ¿De dónde?   a) Where (nationality)

10. ¿A Dónde? means   d)Where (destination)

PRESENT TENSE VERBS TABLE. Please fill in the missing conjugations.

comer	hablar	vivir	tener	ir	ser	estar
Yo como	Yo hablo	Yo vivo	Yo tengo	Yo voy	Yo soy	Yo estoy
Tú comes	Tú hablas	Tú vives	Tú tienes	Tú vas	Tú eres	Tú estás
Él, ella, Ud come	Él, ella, Ud habla	Él vive	Él, ella, Ud tiene	Él, ella, Ud va	Él, ella, Ud es	Él, ella, Ud es

Nosotros comemos	Nosotros hablamos	Nosotros vivimos	Nosotros tenemos	Nosotros vamos	Nosotros somos	Nosotros estamos
Vosotros coméis	Vosotros habláis	Vostotros vivís	Vosotros tenéis	Vosotros váis	Vosotros sóis	Vosotros estáis
Ellos, ellas, Uds comen	Ellos, ellas, Uds hablan	Ellos, ellas, Uds viven	Ellos tienen	Ellos, ellas, Uds van	Ellos, ellas, Uds	Ellos están

PRETERIT. Please fill in the correct conjugations

1. ESTAR a) Juan estuvo b) nosotros estuvimos c) yo estuve
2. QUERER a) tú quisiste b) Jamie y yo quisimos c) vosotros quisisteis
3. TRAER a) Juan y Jorge trajeron b) nosotros trajimos c) el paciente trajo
4. VENIR a) tú viniste b) vosotros vinisteis c) ellos vinieron
5. TENER a) tú tuviste b) Jamie y yo tuvimos c) yo tuve
6. SER a) Juan fue b) nosotros fuimos c) yo fui
7. IR a) Los estudiantes fueron b) nosotros fuimos c) yo fui
8. PODER a) tú pudiste b) yo pude c) ellos pudieron
9. HACER a) tú hiciste b) nosotros hicimos c) ellos hicieron
10. DAR a) tú diste b) yo di c) ellos dieron

IMPERFECT VERB TABLE. Please fill in the missing conjugations.

comer	hablar	vivir	tener	ir	ser	ver
Yo comía	Yo hablaba	Yo vivía	Yo tenía	Yo iba	Yo era	Yo veía
Tú comías	Tú hablabas	Tú vivías	Tú tenías	Tú ibas	Tú eras	Tú veías
Él, ella, Ud comía	Él, ella, Ud hablaba	Él vivía	Él, ella, Ud tenía	Él, ella, Ud iba	Él, ella, Ud era	Él, ella, Ud veía
Nosotros comíamos	Nosotros hablábamos	Nosotros vivíamos	Nosotros teníamos	Nosotros íbamos	Nosotros éramos	Nosotros veíamos
Vosotros comíais	Vosotros hablabáis	Vostotros vivíais	Vosotros teníais	Vosotros ibáis	Vosotros eráis	Vosotros veíais
Ellos, ellas, Uds comían	Ellos, ellas, Uds hablaban	Ellos, ellas, Uds vivían	Ellos, ellas, Uds tenían	Ellos, ellas, Uds iban	Ellos, ellas, Uds eran	Ellos veían

PRETERIT VS IMPERFECT Choose between preterit vs imperfect.

1)  llovía

2) 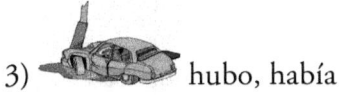 trabajaba

3) 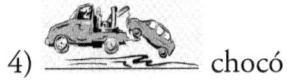 hubo, había

4) 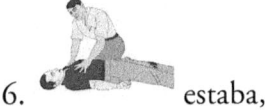 chocó

5. **9-1-1** llamé

6. 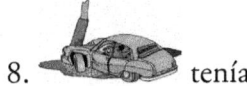 estaba,

7. vino,llevaron

8. tenía

9. 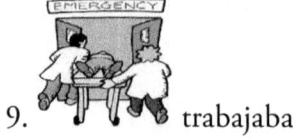 trabajaba

10. 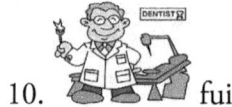 fui

Ser vs estar. Please choose ser or estar in the following sentences.

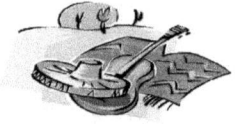

1. está

2. es

3. está

4. es

5. están

6. es

7. es

8. es

9. estoy

10. estamos

www.ingramcontent.com/pod-product-compliance
Lightning Source LLC
Chambersburg PA
CBHW070917220526
45467CB00004B/1436